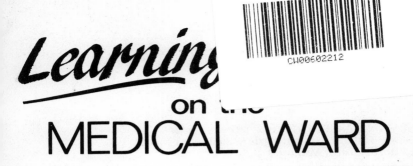

Learning
on the
MEDICAL WARD

Arline Matthews
SRN, DN(Univ. of London)

Ward Sister, Acute Medical Ward, Royal
Hallamshire Hospital, Sheffield

HODDER AND STOUGHTON
LONDON SYDNEY AUCKLAND TORONTO

LEARNING TO CARE SERIES

General Editors

JEAN HEATH, BA, SRN, SCM, CERT ED
National Health Learning Resources Unit,
Sheffield City Polytechnic

SUSAN E NORMAN, SRN, NDNCERT, RNT
Senior Tutor, The Nightingale School, West
Lambeth Health Authority

Titles in this series include:
Learning to Care for Elderly People
L THOMAS
Learning to Care in the Community
P TURTON and J ORR
Learning to Care on the ENT Ward
D STOKES
Learning to Care on the Gynaecology Ward
W SIMONS
Learning to Care on the Psychiatric Ward
M WARD

British Library Cataloguing in Publication Data
Matthews, Arline
    Learning to care on the medical ward. –
    (Learning to care)
    1. Nursing
    I. Title   II. Series
    610.73   RT41

    ISBN 0 340 37062 9

First published 1985
Reprinted 1986, 1988

Typeset in 10/11 pt Trump Medieval by
Rowland Phototypesetting Ltd, Bury St Edmunds, Suffolk

Printed in Great Britain for Hodder and Stoughton Educational,
a division of Hodder and Stoughton Ltd, Mill Road, Dunton Green,
Sevenoaks, Kent, by Richard Clay (The Chaucer Press) Ltd, Bungay, Suffolk

CONTENTS

EDITORS' FOREWORD

In most professions there is a traditional gulf between theory and its practice, and nursing is no exception. The gulf is perpetuated when theory is taught in a theoretical setting and practice is taught by the practitioner.

This inherent gulf has to be bridged by students of nursing, and publication of this series is an attempt to aid such bridge building.

It aims to help relate theory and practice in a meaningful way whilst underlining the importance of the person being cared for.

It aims to introduce students of nursing to some of the more common problems found in each new area of experience in which they will be asked to work.

It aims to de-mystify some of the technical language they will hear, putting it in context, giving it meaning and enabling understanding.

PREFACE

It is a daunting experience to find oneself in unfamiliar surroundings. Most student and pupil nurses new to the medical ward, especially their first nursing experience, will be very apprehensive.

Although there are excellent nursing and medical texts available for reference purposes, there is no book which introduces the nurse to this new experience.

Learning to Care on the Medical Ward attempts to bridge the gap between school of nursing and ward. The approach is basic and simple and aims to introduce the nurse to the type of patients she or he will meet and care for. It illustrates the nursing care those patients will require based on an individual assessment. The nurse can then build on this information through first hand experience, the trained nurses with whom she or he is working, and other texts already available.

I would like to express my sincere thanks to my colleagues who have encouraged and supported me whilst writing this book, and also several student nurses who have given me constructive criticism along the way, and expressed their needs on first coming to a medical ward.

Introduction

Exacerbation
Aggravation of, or
flare-up of a
disease.

**Congestive cardiac
failure** The
output of the heart
is reduced with a
resulting back
pressure which
leads to *oedema* in
the tissues,
congesting them.

Ultrasound A
diagnostic
procedure using
vibrations of the
same nature as
sound waves.
These are passed
through the body
and reflected off
the organ being
investigated. It is
capable of
differentiating
solid from cystic
lesions and can be
used on most
organs as it is a
harmless and
painless procedure.

You are about to work on a ward which is
primarily concerned with the care and treatment of patients with medically orientated
diseases, and the work you are to undertake
will differ from your previous nursing experiences in many ways.

The patients on medical wards rarely have
an operation, although some occasionally do
if, following investigations, surgery is indicated. Medical care does not just involve the
giving of drugs to cure a disease. Many medically orientated diseases are chronic ones,
admission to hospital being primarily to treat
an exacerbation of that disease; for example, a
person with controlled congestive cardiac failure may need admission for treatment of acute
left ventricular failure, or an asthmatic person
may require treatment for an acute asthmatic
attack. Many patients, on discharge home, are
not cured in contrast to what often happens
when surgery is carried out, although their
disease may be brought under control.

Whilst in the ward the patient may need to
undergo a variety of tests and investigations,
some of which will involve you in the collection of specimens or preparation of the patient.
Simple investigations include specimens of
blood, usually taken by the doctor, urine (midstream or 24 hour urine collection), sputum, or
faeces (for occult blood or fat estimation).
Other investigations are more involved, such
as ultrasound scanning of the abdomen and
organs, isotope scans of organs (liver, brain,
etc.) and special X-rays (barium meal, barium
enema, cholecystogram, intravenous pyelo-

Cholecystogram
A special X-ray of the gall-bladder. A radio-opaque dye is taken by mouth and concentrates in the bile.

Venogram A radio-opaque dye is injected into a vein to demonstrate the presence of an abnormality such as a thrombosis.

Chest aspiration
A special needle is passed into the pleural cavity and fluid aspirated. Fluid which collects in the pleural cavity is called a pleural effusion.

Abdominal paracentesis A special needle is passed into the abdominal cavity and fluid allowed to drain away. Fluid collected in the abdominal cavity is called *ascites*.

Bronchoscopy
The examination of the bronchi by the passage of a lighted hollow instrument called a *bronchoscope* via the trachea, under a general anaesthetic.

gram, venogram and angiogram). Samples of various tissue such as lymph gland or kidney may be biopsied, or samples of pleural fluid, cerebrospinal fluid, abdominal fluid or bone marrow aspirated.

The care of patients requires a team approach, involving the patient and his family. The team includes the nurse, doctor, social worker, physiotherapist, speech therapist, occupational therapist, dietician and chaplain, to mention a few. The patients' care must answer their physical, psychological, social and spiritual needs. The nurse should also always think ahead to how the patient and family will cope at home following discharge, e.g. how will the man who has been caring for his demented wife and who has had a cerebrovascular accident (stroke) manage once he is back home, or how will the father of three small children readjust to his daily life following a myocardial infarction (heart attack)? Nursing care and the involvement of other health care workers must be geared to this end.

Members of the caring team

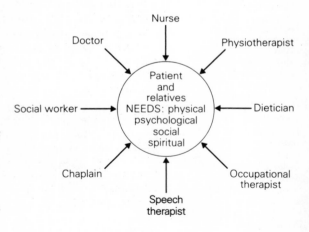

Pressure sore A break in the skin at a pressure point as a result of prolonged pressure.

Deep vein thrombosis The presence of a thrombus in the deep veins of the legs or pelvis. Can complicate injury or bedrest.

Thrombus A clot of blood which blocks the blood vessel in which it is formed, cutting off the blood supply beyond it.

Haematoma A swelling composed of blood suffused into connective tissue.

The majority of patients arrive in a medical ward as emergency admissions, very few from the waiting list. They will therefore be ill or very ill on arrival. Obviously neither the patients nor their families will have had time to prepare for admission to hospital, although some of the patients will have been in hospital before, due to the chronic nature of their disease.

Medical nursing is far less defined than surgical nursing which has well laid-down preoperative and postoperative nursing care. You must remember, however, that although the patients may be very ill, they must move or be moved regularly to prevent developing complications of bedrest, such as chest infection, pressure sores and deep vein thrombosis. Some patients, even when ill, are able to get up and walk around and should be encouraged to do so, and to dress in their day clothes.

The pace on a medical ward may appear to be slower to a nurse who has recently worked on a surgical ward, without the hustle and bustle of patients going to and from the operating theatre. However, medical wards are just as busy but in a different way. There is always something to be done, including sitting and listening, and talking to patients, an aspect of care which is unfortunately often neglected.

Although the patients may be of any age, the majority found here will be in the middle to elderly age range.

A summary of the characteristics of a medical ward:
1 Patients are often chronically ill and are therefore not cured of their disease
2 They rarely have operations
3 The majority of patients are ill-prepared for admission as they are admitted in an emergency
4 They are ill or very ill on admission

5 Care involves meeting the physical, psychological, social and spiritual needs of the patient

6 Misguidedly, the pace of the ward may appear to be 'slower'

7 Patients are often in the middle to elderly age range

Expectations

Let us consider the expectations of you, as a nurse, during your medical secondment:

Your expectations

You will want to:

be accepted as a useful member of the ward nursing team

relate to the patients and be able to talk to them with ease

develop new skills and perfect others

increase your knowledge to gain an understanding of the physical and psychological needs of patients and of the underlying disease process

The patients' expectations

The patients will expect you to:

know what you are doing

be kind, understanding and sympathetic

show empathy

be courteous and helpful to their relatives

not to be familiar

be cheerful and positive but not over-optimistic

communicate in a way they can understand

The ward sister's expectations

The sister or charge-nurse will expect you to:

show that you have commonsense and initiative

act intelligently and thoughtfully

feel free to talk to the patients

be industrious

be cheerful

ask if you are not sure

If in doubt, ask! but remember that there is a right and wrong time to ask questions. Some questions require an immediate answer, such as, 'I've been asked to do this but how do I do it?' Other questions can wait until a more appropriate time if sister is busy, for example, 'It was said in report that Mr Andrews has had a cerebrovascular accident. What does that mean?' In an efficient, caring ward time will always be found later on to answer your question if that moment is not convenient.

Each day you will usually be attached to a senior nurse who will guide you until you gain confidence in yourself and feel secure within the ward. The amount of support and guidance you require will depend on your previous nursing experience. Once you have settled into the ward you will be given more responsibility.

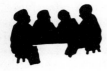

Always remember, however, that different wards are managed differently, depending on the personalities of people making up the ward team, especially that of the ward sister. The specialty also determines how a ward is organised. You need to learn very early in your training to adapt to these various situations and personalities. Try to develop a sensitivity which will enable you to assess the other members of the team and their attitude to you and to nursing and be aware that they also have needs. They have their 'off-days' too. Everyone reacts differently in particularly stressful situations so do make allowances for this, but do not hesitate to ask questions, no matter how silly they may seem to you.

You may feel very apprehensive about your new experience. On arriving at the ward you might feel lost and isolated, especially if you do not know any of the staff, or useless and a 'spare part'.

Demonstrate the commonsense that you already have and, once secure within the ward, use your initiative rather than standing idle, waiting to be told what to do. On the other hand ask the nurse-in-charge or the senior nurse to whom you are responsible what needs to be done next. But you must bear in mind that some senior nurses might think you are over-confident if you do act on your own initiative, so assess the situation carefully when first coming into the ward.

These are some of the more common questions nurses ask themselves:

'How will I know which patients can sit out of bed or walk about?'

Ask the senior nurse to whom you are responsible, or the ward sister.

Refer to the nursing records which should be available and should contain all the information you need to nurse the patient effectively. There should also be a nursing care plan or nursing orders available for each patient. Feel free to look through the nursing notes regularly for they can be very informative, especially if based on a nursing process approach of: assessing patients' nursing needs; planning care to meet these needs; carrying out the planned care; evaluating the effectiveness of the care.

'What should I do if I am asked to do something I have never done before or I do not understand?'

Explain that you are new to nursing or to medical nursing and never be afraid to admit that you do not know.

'How will I react to stress?'

Stress features normally in everyday life and we all react differently to it. Failure to cope depends on many factors but is usually triggered by a minor annoyance. If you feel under stress and cannot cope, ask to talk to sister or a colleague and explain how you feel. She may be able to give you the support and encouragement you need.

'What should I do if a patient collapses and I am the person nearest?'

Ring the emergency alarm bell immediately, or call for help. If this is your first nursing experience you should never be left on your own to cope with such an emergency. This is a problem which worries most nurses and will be discussed more fully in Chapter 8.

'How will I react when I see a dead body for the first time?'

When a patient dies, explain to a senior nurse that you have never seen a body before. A sensitive senior nurse will accompany you to see and touch the body, which will not be as frightening an experience as you might anticipate.

'How will I react if a patient asks me what is wrong with him or if he is going to die?'

Never lie to a patient and never change the subject. If unsure of yourself explain that you are new, or inexperienced, and say that you will fetch a more senior member of the nursing team. Then immediately fetch sister or staff-nurse.

'What do I need to know?'

You must not feel that you have to know everything on your first day on the ward. Although you would obviously like to, it is an impossibility.

To help you to settle into your new environment there are certain things you must know early on in your allocation to enable you to function as a useful member of the ward nursing team. Some wards already have helpful learning objectives. The following set may not be every ward sister's priority but it may help you.

Week I

Layout of the ward – identify sluices, toilets, bathrooms, kitchen, etc.

Names of the ward staff

Names of the patients

Understand the pattern of the patients' and nurses' day

How to use the nurse call system

Fire procedure:
 emergency number to ring
 location of alarm bells
 location of fire extinguishers and hoses
 action to take in case of fire

Cardiac arrest procedure:
 emergency number to ring
 location of equipment
 action that *you* will be expected to take

How to use oxygen and suction equipment

Location of
 procedure manual
 policy manual
 duty rotas
 off-duty request book
 ward learning objectives

How to approach and address patients

Whom to turn to if at all in doubt

The shift system

Mealtimes and location of dining facilities

Week II

Patients' diagnoses – very generally what is wrong with each patient, e.g., Mr Brooks has something wrong with his heart (myocardial infarction), Mrs Chad has something wrong with her red blood cells (anaemia)

Grasp the importance of reporting the slightest change in a patient's condition, e.g., a rise in temperature above normal; bruising in someone with a bleeding disorder; increasing breathlessness in someone with a respiratory disorder

Diagnosis The recognition of disease after consideration of the patient's signs and symptoms.

Anaemia A reduction in the oxygen carrying capacity of the blood, caused by a decrease in the number of circulating red blood cells or haemoglobin, or both.

How to obtain specimens of urine, faeces, sputum, and where to put them

Find your way around the hospital

Locate departments such as haematology, blood bank, chemical pathology, bacteriology, pharmacy, CSSD, X-ray

Understand the principle that *all* drugs, blood and blood products, and intravenous solutions must be checked by a qualified member of the nursing team

How to answer the telephone – remembering the confidentiality of information – but refer all calls to a senior nurse

Understand that patients and relatives will be anxious and frightened

Week III

Having learned generally what is medically wrong with each patient, gain a basic understanding of the disease process to enable you to nurse the patients intelligently

Noticing and appreciating the significance of signs and symptoms so as to anticipate patients' needs

Understand the aim of the nursing care for each patient in relation to their requirements and be able to carry out basic nursing care e.g. bedbath, assisted bath, eye, mouth and catheter care

Use of nursing aids e.g. hoist, sheepskins, cotsides and ripple mattress

Gain some knowledge of the principles and importance of the sterile technique

Subsequent weeks

Understand the importance and reasons for estimating certain physiological measurements, such as hourly pulse, 4 hourly temperature, etc.

Patients' admission procedure

How to use the patients' nursing records

How to obtain blood from the blood bank

How to regulate and change an intravenous infusion

How to give injections – subcutaneous and intramuscular

Assist with a drug round and be aware of some of the more commonly used drugs e.g. Frusemide, a diuretic

During the remainder of the allocation you can now consolidate the experience and knowledge already gained. There will be special procedures which may be performed which you will have an opportunity to observe and discuss with the senior team members e.g. lumbar puncture, bone marrow puncture.

2 Identifying patients' needs

Although some patients come to medical wards as planned (non-urgent) admissions, giving the patient time to prepare for coming into hospital, the majority of the patients are admitted as an emergency (urgent).

The sequence of events will be as follows:

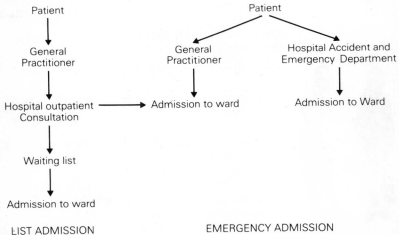

Patient

↓

General Practitioner

↓

Hospital outpatient Consultation ——→ Admission to ward

↓

Waiting list

↓

Admission to ward

LIST ADMISSION

Patient

General Practitioner / Hospital Accident and Emergency Department

↓ ↓

Admission to ward   Admission to Ward

EMERGENCY ADMISSION

Nevertheless, however the patient is admitted, he or she will be frightened and anxious. Some patients will be terrified, but others may feel relieved and more secure once something is being done for them. Remember, too, that the relatives will also be very frightened and apprehensive. Even though it is familiar to you, the ward is strange and frightening to patients and relatives. You may be the first person they encounter, and therefore it is essential that you realise how important your approach is to them; first impressions are often lasting impressions.

It is vital that you understand how the patient and relatives may be feeling, and how they may react to hospitalisation:

| Panic
Anxiety
Fear
Terror
Depression
Insecurity | } caused by | Fear of the unknown
Loss of independence
Inadequate
knowledge
Poor
communication
on the part of
doctors and nurses
i.e. lack of
understanding | } may give
rise to | Weepiness
Questioning/
Non-questioning
Insomnia
Anger/Aggression
Regression/Child-like
behaviour
Rudeness
Attention seeking/
Demanding behaviour
Acceptance/Compliance |

There are several things you can do to ease their tension:

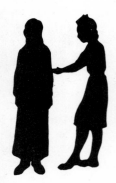

Welcome them with a smile and a kind word
Be courteous
Give them your time even though you may be feeling harassed
Introduce yourself
Introduce the patient to the other patients in the beds nearby
Give relevant information e.g.
    when the doctor is likely to see the patient
    explanation of any equipment in use
    location of locker, wardrobe, etc.
    use of the nurse-call system
    location of toilet, bathroom, dayroom
    mealtimes
    visiting times
    ward routine
Tell the patient what is expected of him or her e.g.
    whether to stay in bed or get up
    whether to change into pyjamas/nightdress
    whether to eat and drink
    if specimens are required (urine, faeces, etc.)
    if dayclothes must be sent home

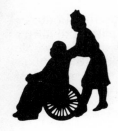

The sort of information you give will depend on how ill the patient is, and whether his or her admission was from the waiting list or as an emergency.

If the patient is not confined to bed a tour of the ward is appreciated as soon as you have time.

Observations and Measurements

It will vary from hospital to hospital whether the patient arrives on the ward in a bed or on a trolley, but once settled into the ward, certain baseline physiological characteristics ought to be measured:

    temperature
    pulse
    respiration rate
    blood pressure
    fluid intake and output
    urinalysis

weight ⎫ may be indicated but will depend on
height ⎬ the state of the patient (this information is sometimes needed to calculate drug dosages)

You will be told how frequently to monitor these measurements. If the patient is very ill these will need to be recorded immediately on arrival so that an assessment of his or her condition may be made.

Thereafter these are recorded at regular intervals, which may be as often as every half-hour or as infrequently as once a day or not at all, depending on the reason for the measurement and the state of health of the patient. This decision will be made either by the nurse-in-charge or by the doctor. Any changes in the recorded measurements must be reported to the senior nurse immediately, who will then decide whether to notify the doctor as a matter of urgency or not.

Physiological measurements should not be made without looking at the patient to form a general assessment. Observation of the whole patient is more important, or equally as important, as the measurements. A great deal of information can be gained from this general observation, such as:

colour of skin
reaction and response
demeanour
interaction with you and others
expression (worried, frightened)
whether drowsy or alert

Medical nursing is based on identifying the nursing needs and problems of patients with medically orientated diseases, planning the care to meet these needs, putting the plan into action and then evaluating the effectiveness of the care given. This is a continuous activity and is commonly known as the *nursing process*.

Henderson's Basic Components of Nursing:

breathe normally

eat and drink adequately

eliminate by all avenues of elimination

move and maintain desired position

sleep and rest

dress and undress

maintain body temperature

keep body clean and well groomed

avoid dangers in the environment

communicate and express emotions, needs and fears

worship according to faith

work at something which gives a sense of accomplishment

play and participate in recreation

learn, discover or satisfy the curiosity

The nursing process is a description of the course of action which takes place when providing individualised care for your patients. It provides a framework for making nursing decisions, setting goals, taking nursing action and measuring nursing effectiveness.

Heath and Law, 1982

Henderson has defined nursing as follows:

Nursing is primarily assisting the individual (sick or well) in the performance of those activities contributing to health, or its recovery (or to a peaceful death) that he would perform unaided if he had the necessary strength, will or knowledge. It is likewise the unique contribution of nursing to help the individual to be independent of such assistance as soon as possible.

The nursing needs and problems you identify after you have gathered together your information will be physical, psychological, spiritual or social. Some of the needs will result from medical intervention. For example, a patient who is incapacitated because of an intravenous infusion will need assistance with personal hygiene and possibly with eating, especially if the free hand does not function adequately (as following a stroke). The intravenous infusion will also require nursing supervision to ensure that it infuses at the required rate and that the cannula remains in position.

Before being able to identify the patient's needs and problems you will require certain information which may be obtained from a variety of sources:

The patient – the nurse talks, listens, observes.

The relatives – the nurse talks, listens, observes. The relatives are often invaluable information sources, especially if the patient is a child, or confused, or unconscious.

The doctor's case-notes (this will avoid the patient being asked the same questions twice)

Other health care workers – social worker, district nurse

Roper's Activities of Living:

maintaining a safe environment

communicating

breathing

eating and drinking

eliminating

personal cleaning and dressing

controlling body temperature

mobilising

working and playing

expressing sexuality

sleeping

dying

By using either Roper's or Henderson's list of activities of daily living as a check list you will have a systematic method of finding out the patient's nursing needs and problems, helping you to achieve an individualised approach to each patient.

The patient's care ought then to be planned according to the identified needs and problems, but you must discuss it with sister or one of the trained nurses on the ward before writing the actual plan. For example:

Mr Jones had a heart attack two days ago and

has come to the ward from the Coronary Care Unit.

Need or problem: Mr Jones is confined to bed and therefore cannot move and may be at risk of developing pressure sores.

Aim of care: to prevent the patient's skin from becoming sore whilst confined to bed.

Plan of care: explain the risk to Mr Jones and the importance of him altering his position at least every two hours whilst in bed. Ensure that he is co-operating. Observe the state of his skin each day.

The plan of care is put into action and the effect of the care evaluated against the desired outcome (the aim). In the case of Mr Jones, evaluation will take place each day – that his skin remains healthy and intact. If the skin begins to redden the plan of care will need reviewing.

To summarise, the nursing process is about:

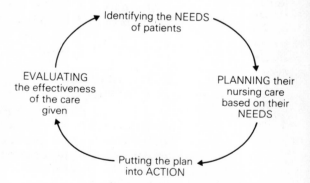

Next you must always consider aspects of care related directly to the disease process e.g. the doctor may require certain physiological measurements to be made by the nurse, specimens of urine, sputum or faeces to be obtained and some patients prepared for special X-rays and investigations. The doctor will require assistance from time to time with technical procedures performed in the ward. Drugs must also be given at certain times as prescribed.

Physiological measurements. These are listed earlier in the chapter, and their frequency may be a nursing decision or a decision made in conjunction with the doctor. You will know how often to record these measurements by consulting the patient's plan of care and the observation charts. The frequency of these measurements will be adjusted by the sister or staff-nurse depending on the patient's improvement or deterioration.

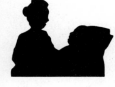

Special X-rays and investigations. The patient may need one or more special X-rays or investigations. The preparation for these will vary from hospital to hospital and you will be advised by the ward sister on what is required. Research has shown that diagnostic tests and procedures are very stressful experiences for patients (Wilson-Barnett, 1978). Each patient will need a full explanation of what to expect prior to, during and after the investigation, as well as details of the preparation required. Patients who are well informed are less anxious, so the time taken is time well spent. They will also want to know from the doctor the results of the test.

Before any special investigation, explain to the patient:

What happens beforehand
Preparation required
What happens during it, and whether there will be any pain or discomfort
What to expect afterwards

Specialised procedures. Some patients may undergo a specialised procedure. In order to know what equipment you ought to prepare before assisting the doctor, you will need to refer to the ward procedure manual and a senior nurse.

It is of paramount importance that, before the procedure commences, the patient has been given a full explanation about what is to happen. As well as assisting during the procedure, it is essential that you observe the patient's reaction, comfort him and allay any anxiety shown. Often the best way to support the patient at such a time is to hold a hand as an act of encouragement and communication. When holding a hand, the nurse may also observe its warmth and colour, steadiness and strength, which are all indicative of changes in the patient's condition.

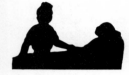

The nurse in the medical ward will need to continually:

Identify the patients' needs and potential problems

Plan and implement care to meet the needs

Support the patient and his or her family

Effectively prepare the patient for planned investigations

Reassure the patient and explain what is to happen to him or her, in order to help to allay anxiety

Continually evaluate care given and revise as indicated

In summary, medical nursing is about:

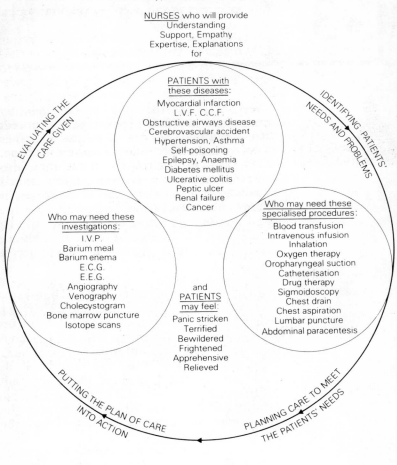

NURSES who will provide
Understanding
Support, Empathy
Expertise, Explanations
for

PATIENTS with
these diseases:

Myocardial infarction
L.V.F. C.C.F.
Obstructive airways disease
Cerebrovascular accident
Hypertension, Asthma
Self-poisoning
Epilepsy, Anaemia
Diabetes mellitus
Ulcerative colitis
Peptic ulcer
Renal failure
Cancer

Who may need these
investigations:

I.V.P.
Barium meal
Barium enema
E.C.G.
E.E.G.
Angiography
Venography
Cholecystogram
Bone marrow puncture
Isotope scans

Who may need these
specialised procedures:

Blood transfusion
Intravenous infusion
Inhalation
Oxygen therapy
Oropharyngeal suction
Catheterisation
Drug therapy
Sigmoidoscopy
Chest drain
Chest aspiration
Lumbar puncture
Abdominal paracentesis

and
PATIENTS
may feel:

Panic stricken
Terrified
Bewildered
Frightened
Apprehensive
Relieved

EVALUATING THE CARE GIVEN

IDENTIFYING PATIENTS' NEEDS AND PROBLEMS

PUTTING THE PLAN OF CARE INTO ACTION

PLANNING CARE TO MEET THE PATIENTS' NEEDS

3 Communication with patients

Everyone needs to talk – patients, relatives, nurses and health care workers. When under stress the need to talk is heightened, and a hospital is an extremely stressful place to be.

The patient or close relative who has been given devastating news will usually want to talk and talk about it – the implications for them, their family and the future – but they will choose with whom they want to talk. The nurse who is feeling under stress or in doubt or upset, under most circumstances will need to talk.

Communication is a two-way process involving interaction both verbal and non-verbal between two or more people. It is a sharing of experience. Information is passed from one person to another which is hopefully received and understood. The information must be interpreted first and must therefore be at the right level, bearing in mind the individual's degree of knowledge, past experience, mental ability and level of intelligence, and also what they may have read or been told by other people.

Do not forget that fear and anxiety usually affect the way in which people are able to interpret what is being communicated to them.

Never talk down to a patient, but never assume that a patient has knowledge, for vital information can get overlooked or misunderstood.

Do not be afraid to go and talk to patients – most patients long for the nurses to talk to them. The need is the same for the young and for the old, for the professional and the unskilled worker. Nurses who become patients also have this need but are unfortunately often neglected in this aspect of their care.

Communication and the receiving of information are often used by patients to measure the standard of care they have received, and this rates highest on the list of complaints made by patients to health authorities. All patients need to know what is wrong with them to a greater or lesser degree, what is going to happen to them, and what they should do.

How do we communicate with our patients?

Meet Mrs White, who has carcinoma of the bowel

HISTORY

Mrs White, a 61 year old widow with two married daughters, was in the acute medical ward being investigated for abdominal pain and change in bowel habit.

A barium enema (see Chapter 6) confirmed a narrowing in the descending colon which was thought to be caused by a carcinoma. Both the physician and surgeon explained the problem and proposed surgical treatment to Mrs White, and that she was to be transferred to the surgical ward later that day.

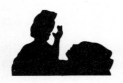

Later in the afternoon the ward sister went to speak to her about the impending surgery and the preparation involved. She asked her how she felt and Mrs White replied that she was very frightened. The sister asked her why she was so frightened. Tears welled up into her eyes and she said that she had never before had an operation or an anaesthetic and this was why she was so frightened.

The sister carefully explained all that was involved between the giving of the premedication and the arrival back on the ward. This seemed to reassure Mrs White and, although still very frightened, her anxiety seemed to lessen a little.

Mrs White's daughters were seen by the doctor when they visited and the planned treatment explained. The sister also saw them and explained why their mother was being transferred to another ward. They wanted to talk to the sister about the possible outcomes following surgery and the fear that the cancer may have spread further. They were reassured that they would be seen again immediately following the operation, and that if the tumour was localised, there was a very good chance of a full recovery. The site of the cancer in the bowel was such that a colostomy was not indicated and this was a great relief to them.

Methods of communication

Communication can be verbal or non-verbal.

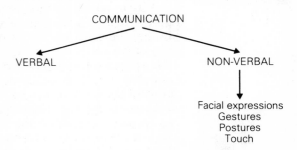

Verbal communication

Verbal communication is the passage of meaningful words from one person to another. The words must be heard and understood so it is essential that the recipient listen and be seen to give attention. There is nothing more off-putting than talking to someone who is not paying attention to you; a patient will soon sense the disinterest.

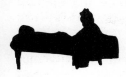

Always
listen
allow patient time to talk, respond, ask questions
pay attention
admit you haven't enough time when busy, but go back later when your work is done

Never
talk at the patient
talk across the patient (too often a temptation when two nurses work together)
make thoughtless comments – these can shatter a patient's trust
appear too busy to talk
use a harsh tone of voice

It is not always essential to sit with the patients in order to communicate with them. In a busy ward communication can take place during the nurse's day-to-day contact with the patient, whilst giving care and carrying out procedures. The important thing is to strike a balance.

Patients and relatives must be kept well informed but will have light-hearted communication with the nurses too.

Research suggests that if patients are given information that enables them to share in their own care, stress is reduced (Boore, 1978). Patients who are made aware of the importance of leg exercises, breathing exercises and moving about in bed to prevent complications arising will usually do so willingly, as it gives them some measure of control, and they are found to be under less stress during hospitalisation.

Poletti's work on stress makes it clear that patients who have relevant information about their treatment and illness which enables them to plan ahead are often less unduly stressed, anxiety is reduced and recovery aided.

Other research suggests that patients are helped if staff are warm, friendly, and informative (Wilson-Barnett, 1979). Hayward's work shows that pre-operative information helps to reduce postoperative pain.

Anticipate questions patients may ask, and when discussing certain aspects of care, give relevant information at the same time, e.g. those who ask:

'Why do I have to drink more?'

'Why can't I eat?'

'Why can't I get up when I want to?'

will probably feel more at ease if they are told the reason why, together with the instruction.

If you are asked questions which you cannot answer, always refer to a trained nurse *immediately*. Never:

change the subject

avert your eyes

ignore the question

feel you must have an answer because you are in uniform

be afraid to say 'I don't know'

Once information has been given to a patient or relative it is usually necessary to test understanding, to invite questions and to reinforce what has been said. The same piece of information may need to be repeated over and over again.

Confidential information

Verbal communication also occurs via the telephone so care must be taken to state who is speaking and only give information received from a senior nurse. Remember that information you acquire in the course of your work is confidential and should not be divulged to other persons either directly or on the telephone. *If in doubt* about this *always* refer to the ward sister or senior nurse.

Non-verbal Communication

Non-verbal communication can be either positive or negative, and can convey many things.

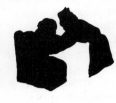

1 Facial expressions. The way a nurse looks will mean much to the patient. A smile is reassuring and conveys compassion and friendliness. A scowl whilst removing a bedpan or changing a colostomy conveys distaste.

When speaking with a person, eye contact is important – it conveys interest. Averting your eyes may give an impression of disinterest or that you may be trying to avoid the truth.

The patient's facial expression may show that the patient is relaxed and trusting, or is anxious, frightened or in pain. Close observation is, therefore, an essential part of good nursing care.

2 Gestures. A nurse who is rushing about may appear to have no time for the patients or to be afraid to talk to them, not that she is busy. Irritability may also demonstrate a lack of care.

The nurse who visits each patient at the beginning of her span of duty is conveying interest and concern.

The patient who snaps fingers or gesticulates wildly may be attempting to cover up anxiety and fear. Those who wring their hands may be frightened whilst those who pace up and down may be anxious or bored.

3 Posture. The position of the body will convey different things to different people. If a nurse confronts a patient with her hands on her hips or arms folded she may convey irritation, impatience or boredom. Nurses slumped over the desk or nurses' station may indicate disinterest in the patients. On the other hand the nurse who stands near to the patient whilst talking or who sits by the bedside will appear interested and aware of the patient's welfare.

Patients who sit slumped in a chair or are unwilling to get out of bed may well be depressed or in pain. Those who hold their head in their hands may be in pain or in despair.

4 *Touch.* Touching rather than speaking can convey much to a patient or relative, especially in a situation where words sound hollow and meaningless. Touch in times of great distress can be comforting, reassuring and gives a sense of support.

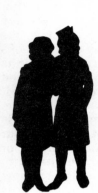

Putting an arm around the shoulder of a bereaved relative usually makes them feel that you understand. Holding the hand of a patient who knows he is dying gives support and comfort and conveys understanding. Patients who are too breathless to speak may gain great comfort from the nurse holding their hand.

Barriers to Communication

Adverse forms of non-verbal communication such as irritability, scowling, hands on hip and gesticulation often inhibit communication. Inattention and lack of eye contact reduces communication between nurse and patient.

If nurses are reluctant to talk and communicate, patients will almost certainly feel uncomfortable, isolated, unwanted and depressed. Good effective communication should lead to a good nurse-patient relationship and certainly helps to determine how the patient feels whilst in hospital. It will also help to preserve the patient's identity in a situation where an individualised approach to patient care is attempted but often thwarted. Unfortunately the hospital is primarily an institution and its organisation is often based on the needs of the staff with the patients being expected to fit into this organisation.

Positive and Negative Expressions of Non-verbal Communication

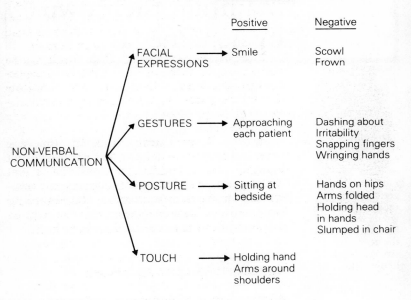

	Positive	Negative
FACIAL EXPRESSIONS	Smile	Scowl Frown
GESTURES	Approaching each patient	Dashing about Irritability Snapping fingers Wringing hands
POSTURE	Sitting at bedside	Hands on hips Arms folded Holding head in hands Slumped in chair
TOUCH	Holding hand Arms around shoulders	

NON-VERBAL COMMUNICATION

4 Nursing patients who are unable to maintain their own hygiene needs

Most of us have a desire to keep ourselves clean and tidy, thus helping us to preserve our dignity.

From your assessment of the patient, by talking with him and his relatives, and observing him, you can ascertain whether the patient will be able to maintain his own cleanliness and comfort or whether nursing intervention is necessary. The patient may not have adequate strength, will or knowledge, or, indeed, strict rest may be enforced, so you need to discuss with a senior nurse the degree of activity the patient is allowed.

NB Bedrest may mean that the patient is not allowed out of bed but may attend to his or her own needs whilst in bed. On the other hand complete bedrest means that everything must be done for the patient by the nurse.

The total hygiene needs of the patient should always be met – cleansing of skin, eyes, nails, mouth, teeth and grooming of the hair. Men will also require a shave.

When independence is lost for whatever reason, frustration often results. When attending to or helping any patient to maintain

Is the patient:

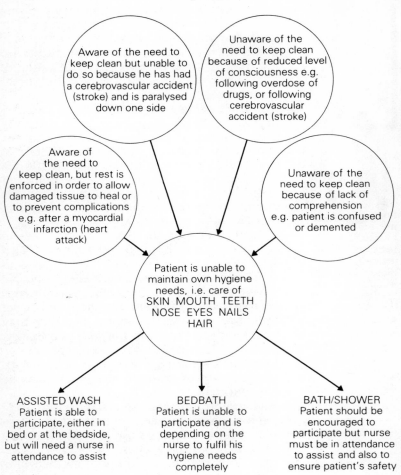

Aware of the need to keep clean but unable to do so because he has had a cerebrovascular accident (stroke) and is paralysed down one side

Unaware of the need to keep clean because of reduced level of consciousness e.g. following overdose of drugs, or following cerebrovascular accident (stroke)

Aware of the need to keep clean, but rest is enforced in order to allow damaged tissue to heal or to prevent complications e.g. after a myocardial infarction (heart attack)

Unaware of the need to keep clean because of lack of comprehension e.g. patient is confused or demented

Patient is unable to maintain own hygiene needs, i.e. care of SKIN MOUTH TEETH NOSE EYES NAILS HAIR

ASSISTED WASH
Patient is able to participate, either in bed or at the bedside, but will need a nurse in attendance to assist

BEDBATH
Patient is unable to participate and is depending on the nurse to fulfil his hygiene needs completely

BATH/SHOWER
Patient should be encouraged to participate but nurse must be in attendance to assist and also to ensure patient's safety

proper hygiene, your approach is of vital importance. If your attitude gives the impression that this is another chore, the patient will feel guilty having to rely on you. On the other hand if you use this time to talk meaningfully with the patient and encourage participation if allowed, it can be beneficial to both patient and nurse.

In some instances this may be an opportunity to involve a close relative in the patient's care, provided that both the patient and the relative – a husband, wife, mother, father, or possibly one of the children – want this. When a patient has previously been looked after at home by the spouse, continuing to include that person in the patient's care is valuable to them both.

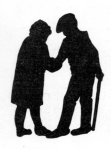

Remember that not every patient needs to be washed from head to toe each day. This depends on:

the patient's wishes. Some elderly people have a bath only once a week, others never. They may be frightened to get in and out of the bath without assistance, and thus may look on their baths in hospital as a luxury. Others may feel it is not necessary.

your assessment of the patient. Is a full bath indicated? For example, the patient may be incontinent.

whether the sister expects it. Unfortunately some sisters still believe patients ought to be bathed every day regardless of their individual needs and wishes.

the other demands of the ward. If the workload is excessive full bathing will not be the most important duty. Top priorities will be mouth care, turning patients and sitting them out, giving fluids, assisting with meals and special treatments, and observing and supporting them.

Whilst washing or bathing the patient, it is essential to observe the state of the skin. Pa-

Physical condition		Mental condition		Incontinent		Activity		Mobility	
Good	4	Alert	4	Not	4	Ambulant	4	Full	4
Fair	3	Apathetic	3	Occasionally	3	Walk/Help	3	Slightly Limited	3
Poor	2	Confused	2	Usually (urine)	2	Chairbound	2	Very Limited	2
Very bad	1	Stuporous	1	Doubly	1	Bedfast	1	Immobile	1

Total the score. If 14 or below patient is at risk of developing pressure sores.

A pressure point is that part of the body in direct contact with a firm surface e.g. bed or chair. If pressure is sustained for any length of time damage to the skin will occur. The skin becomes discoloured and then quickly breaks down. Some patients are more at risk than others.

Pressure points at risk:

Supine patient: sacrum, heels, elbows, scapula area, back of head, knees, spine
Lateral patient: ears, shoulders, hips, knees, ankles
Sitting patient: spine, buttocks

tients confined to bed or chair, especially those with limited movement, are at risk of damaging the skin at the pressure points.

The degree to which any patient is at risk of developing pressure sores can be determined by using an assessment scale devised by Exton-Smith, Norton and McLaren in 1962.

Regular relief of pressure is the only way to reduce the risk of deterioration of the skin at the pressure points. This may be indicated as often as hourly or 3–4 hourly depending upon the individual patient. Whenever possible the patient should be encouraged to assist. As discussed in Chapter 3, by involving patients in their own care, and explaining the importance of altering position at least every 2 hours, whether in bed or in a chair, the risk of sores developing can be reduced.

Aids can be used but should never replace the regular turning of patients. These include: sheepskin rug, sheepskin heel and elbow pads, ripple mattress, net bed, ripple, air, foam and gel cushions, alternating pressure mattress.

It is important to maintain the bedsheets free from wrinkles, crumbs, etc. and the skin should be kept clean and dry. When lifting the patient up it is imperative to avoid dragging the tissues against the bed, so make sure the body is lifted clear. This is possible by using the Australian lifting method (shoulder lift).

Meet Mrs Smith and her daughter

Mrs Smith is an 89 year old lady, who has been reasonably active and maintained good health apart from mild arthritis in her hands and knees. She lives with her single daughter, who is a secretary for a local accountant. Mrs Smith keeps house, cleans, washes and cooks for her daughter.

One morning, on getting up to go to work, Miss Smith found her mother unconscious on the kitchen floor. She immediately called her neighbour and phoned for an ambulance.

Following a thorough examination in the hospital casualty department, the doctor explained to Miss Smith that her mother was unconscious because she had had a stroke – and her condition was critical.

On arrival at the ward, Miss Smith and her mother were met by the ward sister and the nurse assigned to care for Mrs Smith. Whilst two nurses and the porter gently lifted Mrs Smith from the trolley into bed, the sister took Miss Smith into the office as she could see how distressed she was.

Miss Smith immediately burst into tears, bitterly blaming herself for being in bed when her mother collapsed, and for not anticipating that such a thing might happen. The sister comfortingly put her arm around Miss Smith and gently explained that it is not usually possible to anticipate a stroke and that she would not have been able to prevent it. She also went on to say that she was sure that Mrs Smith would not want her daughter to feel guilty and that her mother was probably unaware of the events that occurred at the time she collapsed. Miss Smith seemed calmer and reassured by this and Sister fetched her a cup of tea.

Whilst Miss Smith was drinking the tea the

A stroke is a cerebrovascular accident. This is when the blood supply to part of the brain is cut off, either by a clot of blood (thrombus or embolus), or haemorrhage following rupture of a blood vessel. The degree of incapacity sustained will depend on the part of the brain affected and the amount of brain damaged. Hypertension can cause a cerebrovascular accident.

sister stressed the gravity of the situation, that the stroke was a large one, that Mrs Smith was unconscious and it was highly probable that she would not regain consciousness. Miss Smith asked if her mother was at all aware. Sister explained that it may be possible for the unconscious patient to hear and thus Mrs Smith might be aware of her daughter's presence. She told Miss Smith that she could visit at any time and if she preferred could stay at her bedside. Miss Smith said she would like to stay and found this comforting. After telephoning her neighbour, she was taken by sister to her mother's bedside.

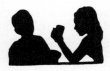

In the ward the nurses had gently positioned Mrs Smith on her side, in order to ensure that her airway remained clear and that she could breathe properly. If placed in the supine position (on the back) there is a very great danger of the tongue falling back and obstructing the trachea when a person is unconscious; therefore all unconscious patients are nursed in the lateral position (on their side) or semi-prone position (upper body chest downwards with head turned to the side and lower body sidewards). Mrs Smith's dentures had already been removed in casualty.

Although she appeared to be deeply unconscious, the nurses talked to Mrs Smith as they positioned her, explaining what they were doing, just in case she was able to hear them. (It is essential to assume that the sense of hearing is retained, and to talk to unconscious patients, explaining and reassuring, whenever attending to them.)

Mrs Smith had vomited a small amount of partly digested food, so the nurses washed her hands and face and put on a clean nightdress, after using a suction catheter to clean her mouth and throat of vomit because of the risk of inhalation and obstructing the trachea or bronchi, which could result in suffocation. She was fed via a nasogastric tube, as unconscious patients must not be fed by mouth due to this dangerous possibility of inhaling food or vomit.

Bed rails or cot sides are used on the beds of unconscious patients for safety reasons, but these were lowered whilst Mrs Smith's daughter was sitting at the bedside to remove the barrier between mother and daughter. In order to offer some privacy, sister drew the curtains around the bed, but not completely isolating Mrs Smith in order that the nurses could continue their observation.

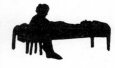

Mrs Smith was a patient in the ward for four days, dying peacefully on the afternoon of the fourth day, with her daughter at her bedside holding her hand. Having assisted the nurses to care for Mrs Smith helped her daughter to begin to come to terms with the sudden illness and death, though she would grieve for a long time.

The following points may be common to all patients following a cerebrovascular accident:

Difficulty in feeding self	Food must be positioned to enable the patient to reach it, and should be cut up. Use of serviettes will help to maintain the patient's dignity and non-slip mat and plate-guard may be helpful.
Contracture of affected limbs which will inhibit recovery of movement	Limbs should be passively moved through full range of movements when turning the patient, and positioned in the natural position both in and out of bed. Refer to physiotherapist.
Difficulty in communicating	Explain all treatments, procedures and plans to patient. Listen carefully and observe for non-verbal forms of communication (especially emotional behaviour brought on by frustration). Use visual aid charts. Refer to speech therapist.

	Frustration at loss of independence	Maintain an optimistic approach and encourage the patient that the aim of care is to gradually enable him or her to regain independence. Encourage participation in activities of daily living with the nurses' help but gradually doing less for patient. Involve relatives. Refer to physiotherapist. Refer to occupational therapist.

CAT scan (computerised axial tomography) of the brain:
X-rays are taken of the brain at different levels, as if slicing the brain across. A computer then produces pictures rather than X-rays. Tumours and haematomas will be shown.

Isotope brain scan:
Radioactive Technetium is given intravenously and taken up by the brain. Potassium perchlorate is given prior to the procedure to prevent the isotope being taken up by the thyroid gland. A scanner is used and will detect the gamma rays which are emitted by the isotope taken up by the brain. The scan will show up space occupying lesions such as a cerebral tumour.

The following points will be common to all unconscious patients:

Airway must be kept clear as it is likely to be obstructed.	Nurse patient on side and maintain position by placing pillow in lumbar region. Remove secretions from mouth or oropharynx if they accumulate.
May develop chest infection due to poor lung expansion	Turn patient regularly to promote better lung expansion.
Likely to develop pressure sores	Keep skin clean and dry and turn 2 hourly from side to side.
May develop a very high temperature which will add to discomfort.	Estimate body temperature 4 hourly (axilla or rectum), and if above 38°C remove blankets, use fan or tepid sponge.
Loss of bladder and bowel control	Catheterise. Give suppositories at regular intervals to avoid constipation.
It is possible that the sense of hearing may be retained.	Talk to patients and never across them. Gently explain all care and reassure.
Is likely to become dehydrated and malnourished	Feeding can be maintained via a nasogastric tube.

Any patient who is unconscious or whose conscious level is depressed and the cause not known, may undergo one or more specific investigations, such as CAT scanning or isotope brain scans.

Complications of Bedrest

Once her needs were identified and nursing care planned accordingly, much of Mrs Smith's care was aimed at preventing the complications of bedrest as all are due to lack of mobility.

All patients confined to bed will be at risk of developing these complications and so the objectives of nursing care will be to prevent their occurrence. This is achieved by recognising that these problems can arise and then planning the appropriate care.

Sites where complications are likely to arise

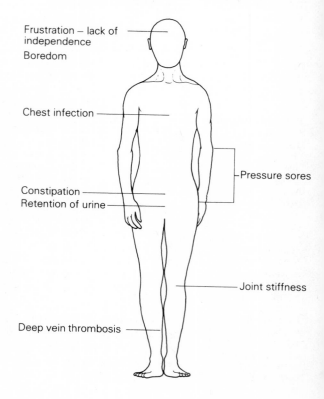

Frustration — lack of independence
Boredom

Chest infection

Pressure sores

Constipation
Retention of urine

Joint stiffness

Deep vein thrombosis

If possible, explain to patients how to help prevent complications; they will feel more involved in their own care and treatment and are more likely to co-operate, thus reducing the incidence of complications.

Common complications:	How the patient can help in prevention:
Pressure sores	Do not sit in one position – lie on sides as well as back. Keep moving in bed.
Chest infection	Take 5–6 deep breaths every hour to fully expand lungs. Discourage smoking.
Constipation	Drink at least 3 pints or 2 litres of fluid a day if not contra-indicated. High fibre diet.
Deep Vein Thrombosis	Do not cross legs. Move legs and wriggle toes at least every hour to stimulate venous return of blood to the heart and prevent stagnation in the veins. Do not rest legs on a pillow.
Joint stiffness	Move and exercise arms and legs.
Frustration and Boredom	Keep informed about treatment and progress. Encourage reading and socialising with other patients.

5 Nursing patients with breathing difficulties

Breathing is essential for life. Respiration occurs both internally and externally to ensure that oxygen arrives where it is needed – in the cells – and that carbon dioxide, a waste product, is excreted.

Some patients are able to breathe without difficulty, others not so easily and others require mechanical assistance. Patients like Mrs Smith (see Chapter 4) are at risk of developing difficulties with their breathing and are, therefore, dependent on the nursing staff to ensure that any difficulty is observed and treated immediately.

Patients who require mechanical assistance may be nursed in special units such as a respiratory unit or intensive care unit, but in some hospitals these patients may be nursed on the acute medical ward.

Bronchitis Inflammation of the bronchioles which may be acute or chronic.

Acute Of sudden onset.

Chronic Present over a long period or re-occurring.

Respiratory or breathing difficulties arise for many reasons. There may be disease of the lower respiratory tract e.g. chronic bronchitis, problems with the respiratory muscles or their associated nerves e.g. poliomyelitis, or the respiratory centre in the brain may be damaged or depressed e.g. drugs such as morphine or barbiturates.

Heart disease, such as left ventricular failure (LVF) and congestive cardiac failure (CCF) will cause difficulty in breathing due to excess fluid in the lungs i.e. the lung tissue becomes waterlogged because the diseased heart is unable to pump efficiently round the body the blood that is returning to its left side from the lungs, and fluid builds up in the lung tissue.

Signs of obstruction of the airway:

noisy breathing
reduced rate of breathing
cyanosis (blue discoloration of the skin)

Oropharyngeal suction is
removing secretions, vomit, etc., from the mouth and oropharynx, by using a suction catheter attached to suction tubing which is attached to a suction machine. This prevents the secretions accumulating in the trachea and obstructing the airway. Ask Sister or Staff Nurse to show you this specialised equipment.

Patients with depression of the respiratory centre in the brain may be unconscious or semi-conscious on admission. It is of paramount importance to observe such patients very closely to ensure that the airway, from mouth to lungs, remains clear and free from obstruction by sputum, secretions, vomit, dentures or the tongue. Therefore, dentures must be removed, and the patient positioned either on one side or in the semi-prone position.

If secretions or vomit block the airway, oropharyngeal suction will be required straightaway – call a senior nurse immediately and *ring the emergency bell*.

Other patients with breathing difficulties will be aware of what is happening around them, but may be afraid because they are not able to breathe properly. This is a very real fear. Most patients are terrified, needing to be constantly reassured that something can and will be done quickly to help them and make it easier for them to breathe.

If treatment is being given, probably by the doctor and a senior nurse, you could sit and hold the patient's hand as this can be very reassuring. You do not necessarily need to talk. The patient will usually be too breathless to talk at this stage.

Different patients will present in different ways, possibly depending on their previous experience. The asthmatic patient, for instance, may have had problems before and overcome them. He or she may think, however, that this occasion might be fatal. It is not unknown for asthmatics to die during an attack of asthma.

It may be the patient's first experience of being unable to breathe, as in a first episode of acute left ventricular failure, and the patient will be terrified, convinced that death is imminent. In this case a calming, reassuring

39

approach is vital, so that the patient realises positive action is being taken.

Do not forget that the relatives are also frightened and extremely worried, needing someone to explain to them what is happening. You will not be able to give them detailed information – the doctor and the senior nurse must do this – but you can explain to them that the patient is being given the appropriate treatment, sit them down and make them a cup of tea.

Once over the initial attack patients may become aware that if they are still finding it difficult to breathe, this will probably affect their lifestyle in the long term and the way in which they cope with the activities of present daily living. This brings an awareness of the need to depend on the nursing team for maintaining hygiene and toilet needs, hydration and nutritional requirements. Severe breathlessness may make eating and drinking difficult; food and drink will need to be within reach of the patient, and the food must be easily digestible.

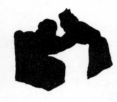

Patients may be unable to do what they did previously – lie comfortably, get up and walk about at will, go to the toilet, maintain their own hygiene needs and enjoy eating and drinking. All these activities now require a lot of effort or may be impossible without nursing help.

This may cause patients much frustration, and they may ask themselves, 'How can I hang on to my independence?' If the respiratory problem is long standing, the patient may have adapted to an accommodating life style, but if the disability worsens, the life style might have to change. This can cause anxiety, anger and frustration or on the other hand, passive acceptance and resignation.

The conscious patient is nursed in the most comfortable position, but should be advised to sit upright supported by pillows and possibly a backrest, or in a high backed chair, all of which will assist expansion of the lungs. Some patients find it easier to breathe by leaning forward over a bedtable, with their arms supported on a pillow. The patient will feel exhausted and need to rest.

The patient may require oxygen. Oxygen should be ordered by the doctor, who will also state the rate at which the oxygen is to be given and the type of appliance to be used.

Oxygen is given when:

1 There is an increased need by the body as in pyrexia
2 The oxygen carrying capacity of the blood is reduced as in anaemia
3 There is a reduction in the amount of oxygen available in the blood as in chronic obstructive airways disease
4 There is decreased cardiac output as in congestive cardiac failure.

Oxygen therapy is the administration of oxygen to a patient at a stated concentration, to increase the oxygen concentration in the blood. There are several appliances that can be used for this purpose e.g. nasal cannulae Ventimask MC mask Look at what is available in your own ward – ask Sister or Staff Nurse to help you.

The patient may be more at ease once the oxygen therapy begins. Some patients however, may experience a sense of panic once the mask is in place and will need to be reassured that this will make them feel less breathless. A full explanation is essential before positioning the mask and commencing the oxygen.

If secretions are present in the bronchi and lungs the use of steam increases humidity and may make it easier for the patient to expectorate; it is given in the form of an inhalation, with or without the addition of a medicant, such as menthol or tincture of benzoin.

Drugs which have a direct effect on the bronchioles, such as Salbutamol, which dilates them, making it easier to breathe, or loosen the secretions, e.g. Airbron, making it easier for the patient to expectorate, may be administered by a nebuliser. This is a device with an oxygen inlet and an outlet to the patient's nose or mouth. Air or oxygen is passed under pressure through the nebuliser. The

Inhalations The inhalation of steam, with or without an added medicament, from a jug or Nelson's inhaler into the respiratory system, in an attempt to loosen secretions. Some drugs are also provided as inhalants which are dispensed in specialised containers.

drug is delivered as a fine spray which is inhaled. Other drugs which act on the respiratory system may be given by mouth or by intravenous injection or infusion.

Meet Mrs Jones admitted with an acute asthmatic attack

Mrs Jones is 36 years old, and has a 15 year old daughter. She has had intermittent admissions to hospital with acute attacks of asthma since she was 21. This time the asthmatic attack was the result of a chest infection which Mrs Jones had had for three days.

After initial treatment in the casualty department Mrs Jones was taken to the medical ward and helped into bed. The nurse assigned to her care welcomed her to the ward, gently told her that she would soon be feeling more comfortable, and ensured that she was well supported with four pillows. The oxygen therapy commenced in casualty was continued.

Mrs Jones' husband sat with her, holding her hand. She found this very reassuring.

As soon as Mrs Jones appeared more relaxed and was breathing more easily, the nurse sat at her bedside and talked to her and her husband in order to assess the patient and identify her nursing needs. Then her plan of care could be made and put into action.

It soon became apparent that Mrs Jones, although relieved at feeling much less breathless, was worrying about her elderly mother. Her mother lived about 10 minutes' walk away but, because of a recent stroke, was housebound and very dependent on her daughter to do her shopping, wash and dress her and clean her flat. No outside help had been needed until now. Mrs Jones felt that she could not expect her daughter to undertake this responsibility as she was currently studying for her end of term exams, and her husband worked shifts.

It was obvious to the nurse that if immediate action was not taken, Mrs Jones' recovery would be hampered by this constant worry. The nurse, therefore, discussed the problem with the ward sister and the following course of action was agreed:

1 Reassure Mrs Jones that the possibility of help for her mother would be looked into immediately.

2 Inform Mr Jones that he could visit at any time to fit in with his shifts.

3 Contact the community nursing service. It was agreed that a community nurse would help Mrs Jones' mother to wash and get dressed each day. This service would continue until Mrs Jones was fully recovered.

4 Contact the hospital social worker. The social worker approached the home help service and the organiser arranged to assess the amount of help needed with shopping, meals and cleaning. The social worker also agreed to visit to make an independent assessment.

5 Ask the ward doctor to contact the General Practitioner. As a result, the General Practitioner said he would visit Mrs Jones' mother as a matter of urgency.

Once these arrangements had been made Mrs Jones was informed of them and she seemed to become more relaxed. Mr Jones said that when he left the hospital he would go to his mother-in-law and explain everything to her.

The next day the oxygen therapy was discontinued as no longer necessary and Mrs Jones was able to sit in a chair, and later in the day, with the help of a nurse, to walk to the toilet. She soon became independent and was discharged home after seven days. The community nurse and the home help continued to care for Mrs Jones' mother for a further month until Mrs Jones was able to resume her support.

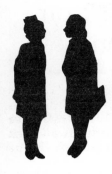

In general, you should remember that any patient with an acute asthmatic attack will need:
specimen of sputum – obtained in a sterile pot, sent to the bacteriology department and any bacteria isolated. The appropriate antibiotics to treat the infection are identified by the bacteriologist.
Antibiotics – drugs aimed at killing or arresting the growth of bacteria.
Chest X-ray
Oxygen therapy
Bronchodilating drugs – drugs which dilate the bronchioles to allow easier inspiration and expiration.

6 Helping patients with hydration, nutrition and elimination

Drinking, eating and elimination are activities of daily living and are basic needs of all individuals.

As the art of nursing is concerned with helping patients to maintain or to meet their basic needs, assisting them with drinking, eating and elimination is an important aspect of nursing care. You will be concerned with all of these as soon as you have contact with the patients in the acute medical ward, or any type of ward.

Although hydration, nutrition and elimination are all interlinked, here they will be considered separately.

Hydration

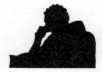

In health most people are able to maintain an adequate intake of fluids for the proper functioning of the body, and the sensation of thirst indicates that more fluid is needed. The normal daily fluid requirement is 2000–2500 ml. In illness however, there might be many reasons for a variation in the fluid requirement of an individual.

The fluid requirement may be normal but the patient may not be able to maintain this for himself due to a variety of reasons:
  damage to the brain may result in the patient being unable to translate the sensation

Haemorrhage
Bleeding from burst
blood vessels. May
be profuse.

of thirst e.g. with damage due to a tumour,
blood clot or haemorrhage.

a disability may make it physically impossible for the patient to get a drink, especially if it is placed out of reach e.g. following a cerebrovascular accident

loss of consciousness

sore mouth

loss of the swallowing reflex

The fluid requirement may need to be in excess of normal due to:

high temperature (excess fluid lost due to sweating)

vomiting and/or diarrhoea, causing excessive fluid loss

excessive urine output

dehydration

Self-poisoning
The intentional
ingestion of
poisons e.g. drugs
or noxious
substances, in an
attempt to commit
suicide, to attract
attention or as a cry
for help.

there may be a need to increase the renal output in order to flush out poisons or toxic waste products from the body e.g. after a patient has taken an overdose of drugs

The fluid requirement may need to be less than normal due to:

malfunction of the kidneys which are not able to remove fluid adequately

severe heart failure in which fluid is retained in the tissues

in preparation for certain tests and investigations, especially on the gastrointestinal or renal systems.

Renal failure   The
failure of the
kidneys to excrete
waste products
from the body. Can
be acute or chronic,
and reversible, or
fatal without a
kidney transplant.

If fluid requirement is restricted it may involve nil orally or as little as 30 ml water every hour.

If the patient is not able to obtain fluids without help and is dependent on other people, he or she may feel thirsty. This will also occur with patients in whom the fluid intake is restricted. Therefore, always remember what it is like to feel thirsty, and ensure that drinks are to hand or that patients who need help are given the necessary assistance. Remember that dribbling is embarrassing and thus the use of a beaker or feeding cup may be indicated, but, on the other hand a feeder may, to many patients, be undignified. Also remember to protect the patient's clothing.

If fluid intake is inadequate, dehydration may result and this may be disastrous for the patient.

Those patients who have a restriction on their fluid intake may not understand why they are not allowed to drink freely:

'Why can't I drink more, nurse?'

'Why can't I drink what I want to?'

Careful explanation is essential and may need to be repeated often. Frequently moistening the patients' lips and encouraging them to suck boiled sweets – if allowed – stimulate the secretion of saliva and help ease the discomfort.

Patients requiring a fluid intake in excess of normal may well keep asking:

'Why do I have to drink so much?'

'I cannot possibly drink more.'

'The tea, water and coffee don't taste the same as at home.'

'All this drinking is making me want to keep going to the toilet.'

Ingenuity on the part of the nurse and much encouragement for the patient is needed here. This will include:

A variety of drinks

Assessing likes and dislikes

Involving family and friends

Involving the patient in recording his or her fluid intake

Careful measuring and recording is required of all fluid taken in and all fluid passed from patients having restricted fluids or excessive fluids, and those with renal or possible renal problems. This is known as recording the patient's intake and output, or fluid balance.

Fluid intake:

fluid taken orally
fluid given intravenously
fluid given rectally
fluid given via a nasogastric tube

Fluid output:

urine
diarrhoea
vomit
fluid drained or aspirated from any tube
fluid lost through a fistula

Remember to measure and record any fluid that the relatives may give the patient and the time at which it was given. This will mean explaining to them that all fluid has to be recorded, as their involvement is essential if accuracy is to be maintained.

Patients who are not able to take an adequate amount of fluid orally, those in which potassium chloride or special drugs, such as certain antibiotics, need to be given directly into the venous system, and those requiring blood or blood products, will have an intravenous infusion in progress. This is often referred to as a 'drip'.

In most hospitals the setting up of an intravenous infusion is undertaken by the doctor assisted by a nurse. The changing of the bags of fluid is performed by the nurse, following the doctor's written instructions.

Intravenous Infusion:

The continuous administration of fluid, with or without the addition of drugs, into the venous system e.g. normal saline
dextrose with saline
dextrose
blood
blood products e.g. plasma, platelets

Meet Mr Green who has a peptic ulcer

HISTORY

Mr Green is a 45 year old man who is known to have an ulcer in his duodenum. One evening, whilst at home with his wife watching television, he suddenly feels dizzy and sick, and vomits a large amount of blood (haematemesis). He feels cold and clammy, and then has his bowels open. The stool is black and tarry (melaena).

Both Mr and Mrs Green are very frightened by what has happened, and Mrs Green rings for the doctor immediately. The doctor arrives quickly, examines Mr Green and arranges his admission to hospital straightaway.

On arrival at the ward Mr Green is very cold and clammy, his blood pressure is 90/48 mm Hg and his pulse 132 beats per minute. He is pale, restless and frightened. These observations all indicate a shocked patient resulting from a sudden loss of blood.

Peptic ulcer An ulcer arising in the mucous membrane in the stomach, duodenum or at the lower end of the oesophagus.

Tachycardia A heart rate of over 100 beats per minute.

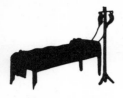

The nurse responsible for Mr Green's care reassures him that immediate action is to be taken and that soon he should be feeling more comfortable. She helps the doctor to site an intravenous infusion and Mr Green is given normal saline and then plasma until blood is available for blood transfusion. (Blood from the Blood Transfusion Service has to be matched with a specimen of blood from Mr Green.)

The nurse measures and records all urine, vomit and stools passed by Mr Green, and is careful to describe the nature of the vomit and the stools in the nursing records and on the relevant observation charts. She also records all fluid given intravenously to Mr Green.

All this information will be used by the doctor when evaluating Mr Green's progress and treatment, therefore accuracy in record keeping is essential.

During this time the ward sister, having assessed Mr Green's condition and ensured that his immediate needs are being met, is talking to Mrs Green, explaining to her all that is being done for her husband, and reassuring her that the doctor will explain to her the medical facts as soon as he is free. The sister also ascertains where Mrs Green can be contacted in case her husband's condition deteriorates, and obtains a reliable phone number. She ensures that Mrs Green has someone to fetch her home once she has seen her husband.

Mr Green vomits a further 200 ml of blood and passes another small melaena stool. The vomiting then subsides.

In order to confirm the cause and site of the bleeding the doctor decides to perform a gastroscopy. The patient must be starved prior to the procedure. If an abnormality is noted a biopsy may be taken.

A biopsy is the removal of a piece of tissue which is then sent to the pathology laboratory where its nature is determined by the pathologist e.g. benign ulcer, inflammation, carcinoma, etc.

Gastroscopy is the passage of a flexible lighted instrument via the oesophagus into the stomach, to enable the doctor to examine the lower end of the oesophagus, stomach, pylorus and duodenum for any abnormality such as ulceration, carcinoma or erosion of the mucosa. Prior to the procedure the throat is usually sprayed with local anaesthetic and the patient given a muscle relaxant drug. Following the procedure the patient is advised not to eat or drink until the swallowing reflex returns i.e. until the effects of the local anaesthetic have worn off.

A barium meal is a special X-ray procedure which involves the patient swallowing a radio-opaque substance, barium, following which X-rays are taken. The lower end of the oesophagus, the stomach and duodenum are outlined and abnormalities, such as ulcers, oesophageal varices or carcinoma, can be demonstrated. The patient must be starved for 4 hours prior to the procedure to ensure that the stomach and duodenum are empty.

Mr Green is allowed small amounts of fluid to drink, the amount gradually increasing over the next 24 hours and then he commences a very light diet.

Sometimes a barium meal may be arranged to ascertain the cause of haematemesis and melaena.

Nutrition

In health people may or may not maintain their correct nutritional requirements. Those people who take in amounts of food over and above their bodily requirements may be overweight or obese, whereas those who have an inadequate intake may be underweight.

A healthy nutritional intake includes the correct amount of carbohydrate, fat, protein, vitamins and minerals for the individual.

Liver failure The failure of the liver, due to a variety of causes, to carry out its normal functions. Usually it is a chronic condition which may be controlled but not cured. Certain drugs or poisons may cause reversible acute liver failure.

In illness the nutritional requirements for the individual may be normal, but the patient may not be able to maintain his intake without assistance. On the other hand the nutritional requirements may be in excess of, or less than, normal. Individual components of a normal diet may be restricted in various diseases, e.g. protein in renal or liver failure, carbohydrate in diabetes mellitus, or fat in gallbladder disease.

Nurses must be involved in the serving of patients' meals, even if meals come to the ward marked for the individual patient, so that they know what is required and can suggest substitutes. If a menu system is in use, some patients may need the assistance of the nurse to complete their menu cards.

When assisting with meals remember that sometimes food will have to be cut up, some patients will need help with feeding and *all meals must be placed within reach.*

It is essential to always remember what it must feel like to be hungry but not able to get to your food, or to be unable to cut it up. It is degrading to be clumsy when eating and this should be taken into account when assisting the patient, care being taken to minimise embarrassment and to protect the patient's clothing by the proper use of napkins.

Nutritional Requirement – normal intake, but patient not able to maintain unaided because:	Nutritional Requirement – in excess of normal because of:	Nutritional Requirement – less than normal because of:
↓	↓	↓
Not able to recognise hunger Not able to feed self because of confusion or disability Unconscious Sore mouth Loss of swallowing reflex	Anorexia, nausea Vomiting Diarrhoea Excess cell breakdown e.g. in malignant disease and during cytotoxic chemotherapy or radiotherapy	Obesity Preparation for certain tests and investigations

Nasogastric Tube Feeding is the passage of fluid of a predetermined calorific and food value, into the stomach, via a tube passed through the nose, oesophagus and then into the stomach.

Remember, also, that to need to be fed can be most undignified.

Patients with loss of the swallowing reflex or who are unconscious may need to be fed via a nasogastric tube. The feeds may be prepared in the ward kitchen but usually the dietician is involved and the feeds are prepared centrally and sent to the ward from the diet kitchen.

Parenteral Feeding is the administration of a patient's nutritional requirements by the intravenous route, the deep veins, as opposed to the superficial veins, being used. The total calorific and vitamin requirements are given over a period of 24 hours.

It may be considered desirable in some cases to feed a patient by the parenteral route.

Elimination

Elimination is the process by which the normal healthy body gets rid of waste products and excess fluid.

In health the average person passes approximately 1500 ml of urine every 24 hours and empties the bowels at fairly regular intervals, varying from twice a day to once every 3 or 4 days. It is important to know the individual patient's normal habit, as changes of environment, level of activity or diet often affect bowel habits.

Under normal circumstances elimination is a very private affair for the individual, and in hospital every effort must be made to maintain this privacy. Always remember that to have to rely on another person to assist with going to the toilet is embarrassing.

When giving bedpans, urinals, or a commode ensure that privacy is maintained and, if possible, leave the patient unless unsafe to do so, with a bell to hand.

Using a bedpan may cause excessive strain which should be avoided whenever possible. The patient who has had a myocardial infarction or subarachnoid haemorrhage may put less strain on the heart or the cerebral blood vessels if allowed to use the commode with the nurse's assistance rather than perch on a bedpan.

Encourage the use of the commode or, better still, take the patient to the toilet, on a wheelchair if he or she is not able to walk. If in doubt consult the care plan or ask a senior nurse.

Taking the patient to the toilet may take more time, especially if the patient has a disability such as severe rheumatoid arthritis, but

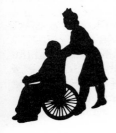

Diabetes mellitus
The partial or complete failure of the pancreas to produce insulin, resulting in the incomplete utilisation of carbohydrate. It is treated with dietary restriction of carbohydrate with or without the addition of insulin or oral hypoglycaemic agents.

Haematuria The presence of blood in the urine.

Urinary Catheterisation is the passing of a catheter, under aseptic conditions, into the bladder. In the case of loss of bladder control it is retained by means of a small balloon, to allow continuous drainage of urine.

the effort is worthwhile for most patients and it also encourages independence.

On admission to hospital all patients should have their urine tested to eliminate any abnormalities which might indicate underlying disease, e.g. presence of glucose may indicate diabetes mellitus, presence of protein may indicate renal disease.

Test the urine as soon as possible. Do not forget to tell the patient that a specimen is required and provide him or her with the appropriate container with instructions of what to do with it once used. Having tested the urine do not forget to chart it – ask sister or staff nurse where to record your findings.

For some patients each specimen of urine which they pass must be tested, for others several specimens a day, as with diabetic patients, and for others once daily as with those on certain drugs such as steroids (which may cause glucose in the urine) or anticoagulants (which may cause blood in the urine). The results are usually entered on a special chart at the patient's bedside or in the nursing notes.

In illness elimination may be a problem. There may be loss of bladder or bowel control resulting in incontinence of urine or faeces, or both. On the other hand there may be an inability by the patient to empty either the bladder or the bowel.

Some patients who have lost control of their bladder function may need to be catheterised. Catheterisation is performed by a skilled person under aseptic conditions in total privacy, following explanation to the patient. If not performed properly it carries the risk of damage or infection to the urinary tract.

If catheterisation is contraindicated and the patient is incontinent of urine, retraining of the bladder is essential. This involves sitting the patient on a bedpan or commode or taking him to the toilet at regular intervals, as often

Empathy Putting oneself totally in the position of another and experiencing how that other person feels.

as every hour or two hours. The use of special incontinence pads and pants may also be indicated.

Patients who are incontinent will be most embarrassed and must never be scolded. Try to imagine what it feels like not to be able to control your bladder, to lie in a wet bed or not be able to get to the lavatory without help. It is most humiliating and empathising with the patient will help to restore self-confidence and self-esteem.

To be incontinent of faeces is even more humiliating and should be dealt with tactfully and sympathetically and with the minimum of fuss. Some patients may have more confidence if, when there is a tendency towards incontinence, they are nursed on an incontinent pad as they feel that the bed is protected. It is, however, important to reassure them that it is no problem to change the bed when necessary.

Semiconscious patients may become very restless when incontinent, and confused patients often try to get out of bed. Patients who are unconscious or confused should have their bladder and bowel action recorded in order that constipation or urinary retention does not go unnoticed.

Diarrhoea is the passing of frequent loose stools.

Causes in a medical ward:
Reaction to certain drugs e.g. antibiotics
Food poisoning
Infection in the bowel
Ulcerative colitis
Crohn's disease
Bleeding from stomach or duodenum
Cancer of the large bowel
Diverticulitis
Malabsorption
Faecal impaction with false diarrhoea

Diarrhoea is a very embarrassing condition, especially for the patient who is confined to bed. It is often associated with abdominal pain and can be a very miserable occurrence.

Efficient removal of bedpans or commodes, without chastisement and with a minimum of fuss, helps to reduce embarrassment for the patient.

If diarrhoea is a problem the nature and frequency of the stools should be recorded on a special chart or in the nursing notes, and the doctor informed of any worsening of the diarrhoea. It is cured by treating or removing the cause and giving anti-diarrhoea preparations such as kaolin mixture or codeine phosphate.

Constipation is uncomfortable and often very painful, causing patients a lot of unnecessary suffering, frustration and embarrassment. In many cases it can be avoided by good nursing care.

Good observation of the patient and careful monitoring of each bowel action, especially for patients who are vague or forgetful, are essential.

Do not forget that some patients who are fully independent may be embarrassed to say that they have not had their bowels opened for several days, so it is essential for the nurse to broach the subject.

The administration of aperients before the patient becomes uncomfortable often prevents constipation, but consultation with the patient is essential. How the patient feels and the normal bowel habit need to be taken into consideration.

The action to be taken and the type of suppositories or enemas to be used will be decided by the sister or staff nurse in consultation with the doctor, and you will need supervision by a trained nurse if you are included in resolving the problem.

Constipation is difficulty or inability to evacuate the bowel

Causes in a medical ward:
Reaction to certain drugs e.g. opiates
Change of environment
Reduced activity
Reduced roughage intake
Cancer of the large bowel

Methods of dealing with constipation:

high roughage diet
adequate fluids
increased activity
aperients
suppositories
enemas
rectal washouts
manual evacuation

HISTORY

Meet Mrs Johnson who has Ulcerative Colitis

Mrs Johnson is a 28 year old mother of two children aged 5 and 2 years. She has had diarrhoea for 3 weeks, passing up to 12 very loose stools a day. On admission she looks pale and thin and is obviously very tired, having had disturbed nights since the diarrhoea began.

Arriving at the ward with her husband, Mrs Johnson is very worried about her health and also extremely upset and anxious because she has not been separated from her children before. She is frightened as, apart from the birth of her two children, she has never been in hospital. A thoughtless neighbour has also mentioned an operation to her and this has heightened her fear and anxiety.

This information was volunteered straightaway by Mr Johnson and the ward sister immediately identified the following problem:

Acute anxiety and fear due to:
   separation from children
   fear of hospitals
   sudden onset of illness in an otherwise healthy adult
   fear of possible surgery

How would you deal with this?

NURSING CARE

The action taken was as follows:
1   Separation from children
The sister ascertained that they were being cared for. The grandparents who live next door and with whom the children get on very well, are looking after them whilst their father is at work. The sister emphasises to Mr and Mrs Johnson that the children may visit their mother as regularly as possible, except during patients' rest hour.
2   Fear of hospitals
Mrs Johnson was introduced to the patients in her cubicle, and taken on a tour of the ward. Uniforms, special equipment and ward routine were explained. She was told that she could wear her day clothes if she wished.
3   Worry about sudden illness

Ulcerative colitis A severe inflammation of the rectum and large intestine. It is a chronic condition of unknown cause.

It was explained that Mrs Johnson was thought to have a condition called ulcerative colitis (inflammation of the bowel). It was hoped to confirm this with some X-rays and bowel investigations. Once confirmed, treatment would be started which should control the diarrhoea and make her feel much better, so that she could continue to lead a normal life.

4   Fear of surgery

Mrs Johnson was reassured that her illness would be treated with drugs and dietary control and that surgery would not be contemplated unless she failed to respond to conservative treatment.

The other major problem was of diarrhoea and weight loss.

How would you deal with this?

The following action was taken:

1   Bed located near a toilet and the toilet pointed out to Mrs Johnson.

2   Explanation of the need to observe the nature and frequency of stools and the provision of a supply of named bedpans and covers. Observation of stools for: volume, colour, consistency, frequency i.e. date & time, presence of mucus, presence of blood, recorded on a special chart at the bedside and/or in the nursing records.

3   Explanation of the need to take only fluids in order to rest the bowel. Nourishing fluids such as Complan, Buildup and special high calorie drinks with added vitamins would be provided in place of solid food.

4   The importance of rest was stressed and that lying down for long periods is acceptable.

Bowel investigations may be performed before a diagnosis of ulcerative colitis is made, such as faecal analysis, sigmoidoscopy, colonoscopy and barium enema.

Faeces for occult blood is the collection of three consecutive specimens of faeces (a small portion of the stool) which is sent to chemical pathology where the presence of any blood, not obvious to the naked eye, is estimated. During the collection most physicians prefer the patient to have a diet free from red meat.

Faecal fat collection is the collection of all stools over a 3 or 5 day period, in special large containers. The amount of fat present is estimated by the clinical pathologist. During the collection a normal diet is usually given. The result will indicate whether absorption from the small bowel is defective.

Sigmoidoscopy is the passage of a rigid lighted instrument into the rectum and sigmoid colon in order to examine their mucosa. Some doctors prefer the patient to have a disposable enema prior to the procedure. Haemorrhoids, polyps, carcinoma or colitis may be diagnosed.

Colonoscopy is the passage of a lighted, flexible instrument into the colon via the rectum and sigmoid colon. The large bowel is examined and biopsies may be taken. Conditions such as ulcerative colitis, diverticulitis, polyps or carcinoma may be diagnosed. Prior to the procedure the large bowel is emptied by giving aperients and a fluid diet.

Barium enema is the introduction of barium, a radio-opaque liquid, into the large bowel as an enema. An empty colon is essential and aperients, enemas and a fluid diet are given prior to the procedure. Ulcerative colitis, polyps, diverticulitis or carcinoma of the colon may be diagnosed.

Other investigations may be indicated for patients with problems of the bladder including urine analysis and intravenous pyelogram.

Midstream specimen of urine (MSU) is the collection of a specimen of urine once the flow of urine has begun. The genital area is cleaned first to prevent contamination of the specimen by organisms outside the urinary tract.

24 Hour Collection of Urine is the collection of all urine passed by a patient in a 24 hour period. The urine passed at the commencement of the collection is discarded and that passed on completion of the 24 hours is saved. The clinical pathologist can estimate presence of urea, electrolytes, protein, etc. and the results are used to estimate renal function, endocrine function, etc.

Intravenous pyelogram (IVP) is an X-ray of the renal tract. A radio-opaque fluid is injected into the venous circulation and as it is excreted through the kidneys X-rays are taken of the kidneys, ureters and bladder. Abnormalities in this system will be highlighted. It is essential that the bowel is free of faeces and gas as this will obscure the X-rays. Aperients and suppositories are given and food and fluids restricted on the day of X-ray.

7 Protecting patients from harm and aiding independence

Consider the following: how does it feel to be dependent on others?

How would you feel if:

You were not able to go to the toilet when you wanted to?

You were not able to get a drink when you wanted one?

You were not able to cut up and eat your food?

You were not able to get up, have a wash, clean your teeth, comb your hair and cut your nails?

You were not able to dress or undress yourself?

You were not able to go to the telephone?

You were not able to go home with your family or friends?

You were not able to talk and converse as you would like?

You were unable to get warm, or cool, without assistance?

Nursing is assisting the individual in any of these activities he or she cannot perform alone. It is also helping the patient back to independence in all, or some of these aspects of daily living. Independence gives self-respect, so it is important for all patients to achieve as great a degree of independence as possible.

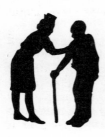

There is a tendency to overprotect patients and not to encourage them to do enough for themselves. This is often due to conflicts between:

Time required and time available
Encouraging independence but ensuring safety

It is often quicker and safer for the nurse to do it. If a patient is actively seeking independence the nurse may be in a dilemma. Should I let the patient 'go it alone'? Here the sister or trained nurse must give the necessary guidance.

Some aids to mobility and independence:

Walking
gutter frame – has wheels and arm supports – is elbow high
rollator frame – has wheels – is hand high
zimmer frame – no wheels – is hand high
tripod – three pronged walking stick
quadrapod – four pronged walking stick
crutches
walking stick

Eating
plate guard – clips on side of plate so that food is pushed against it and stops it falling off plate
non-slip mat
cutlery with built up handles – to enable firmer grip

Dressing
zip aid
stocking aid
long-handled shoe horn
elastic shoe laces
use of velcro on garments

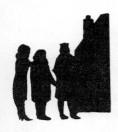

Other health care professionals are involved in the rehabilitation of patients (see Chapter 1), including the physiotherapist, occupational therapist and speech therapist. When it is apparent that the patient will be able to return home the district nurse and social worker are also involved.

Patients should be encouraged to get dressed whenever possible – this not only helps in their rehabilitation but is a morale booster for any patient. Some patients – those who are confused and at risk of coming to harm – may need the use of special aids in an attempt to avoid injury. Before these are used, however, it is important to ascertain whether the nurse can do anything to reduce confusion and whether the use of an aid may aggravate the patient and increase the risk of injury. For example, some patients may become more agitated if safety rails are used and they may attempt to climb over them. If it is an adjustable-height bed it may be safer to put it to its lowest level without the safety rails.

Some factors which can increase mental confusion in patients but which may be corrected by the observant nurse:

The need to micturate or defaecate, or constipation
Lying in a wet bed
Being too hot or too cold
Being afraid
Being lonely
Not understanding what is happening to self
Hunger and thirst
Certain drugs
Darkness and unfamiliar surroundings
Reduction of oxygen to brain (hypoxia is one of the commonest causes of confusion at night, especially with bronchopneumonia)

Aids used to protect patient:

adjustable-height bed
safety rails/cot sides
chairs with fixed tables
tilt-back chairs

Close observation of confused patients is extremely important, and even if an aid for protection is used, this does not diminish the need to continue to observe the patient.

Some medical causes of acute confusional toxic states:

Infection with high temperature
Certain drugs e.g. Lignocaine IV, Morphine
Drug abuse and withdrawal
Alcohol abuse and withdrawal
Intracerebral lesions e.g. tumour, clot, haemorrhage

Patients may be admitted to the ward following an epileptic fit, or may have a fit whilst a patient. This can be a very frightening experience for the patient, the other patients and for the nurse, especially if they have never witnessed an epileptic fit before. During a fit the patient is at risk of harming himself and the nurse has a responsibility to try to prevent this.

Epilepsy is the production of excessive electrical stimuli by the brain cells resulting in uncontrolled movements of the muscles of the body, which may either affect the whole body (grand mal), or a small part of the body (focal fit).

Commonly known as fits, they can be caused by tumours, a blood clot, certain poisons such as drugs or alcohol, or following injury or surgery to the brain. They can also be idiopathic (of no known cause).

Epileptic patients should be encouraged to lead as normal a life as possible, and when in the ward this means allowing them to be independent. There is no reason why they should not dress in their day clothes but this will depend on ward policy.

The main responsibility of the nurse is to observe for any epileptic fits, and if one does occur to take the following action:

Stay with the patient

Protect the patient from harming self but allowing the fit to run its course (do *not* forcibly restrain the patient)

Maintain a clear airway

Observe and time the length of the fit and note:

    which limbs are affected

    how the limbs are affected

    whether the jaw is clenched

    whether the tongue is bitten

    whether there is any incontinence

Do not try to move the patient during the fit

After the fit put the patient into bed on his or her side to ensure a clear airway and allow to sleep.

Observe closely for further fits.

Reassure the patient as awareness is registered.

If a patient has a fit and is not known to be an epileptic, he or she must be fully investigated to exclude a treatable cause. One of the most important investigations is an electro-encephalogram (EEG).

Electroencephalography (EEG) involves attaching electrodes to the scalp and recording the electrical activity generated by the brain cells. It will help to diagnose the type of epilepsy and aid the treatment.

Apart from explaining to the patient what is involved, there is no special preparation except that the hair should be washed to remove any grease. The hair may also need washing afterwards to remove the jelly used to obtain good electrode contact.

Once diagnosed and a cause excluded, epilepsy is treated with drugs to reduce the excitability of the nerves and reduce the number of fits e.g. Phenytoin.

Advice given to epileptic patients on discharge from hospital:

1   Try to lead as normal a life as possible but avoid activities of a risky nature e.g. swimming, climbing.
2   Take the tablets at the prescribed times and never miss a dose.
3   Do not work with heavy machinery – this may need the involvement of the social worker and Disablement Resettlement Officer (DRO) to help the patient find more suitable employment.
4   If the holder of a driving licence inform the licensing authority straightaway.
5   Involve the family, instructing them what action to take in the event of a fit, but also encouraging them to allow the patient to lead as normal a life as possible.

HISTORY

Meet Mrs Davis who has had a Subarachnoid Haemorrhage

Mrs Davis is 42 years old, and teaches geography at the local senior school. She has a 15 year old daughter, Sarah, and a 19 year old son, Paul.

Following one teaching session Mrs Davis complained of a sudden violent headache, associated stiffness and pain in her neck and a sensitivity to light (photophobia). Her colleagues encouraged her to lie down but the pain quickly worsened and she began to feel very sick. Mrs Davis was obviously very distressed so they contacted her husband who took her home by car. There he contacted the family doctor who immediately diagnosed a subarachnoid haemorrhage and arranged for her immediate admission to hospital.

A subarachnoid haemorrhage is rupture of a cerebral blood vessel, resulting in bleeding into the subarachnoid space of the brain and spinal cord (between the pia mater and the arachnoid mater). There is usually a congenital abnormality at the site of damage, either an aneurysm or an arteriovenous malformation. It may result in paralysis, unconsciousness or death.

Congenital abnormality
An abnormality present at birth but not inherited.

Arteriovenous malformation
A congenital abnormality of part of the cerebral circulation, where there is an unstable network of arteries and veins.

The Circle of Willis – Cerebral Circulation (blood supply to the brain)

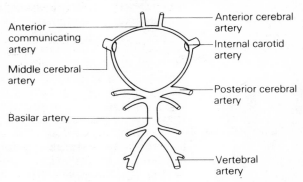

The admitting doctor agreed with the family doctor's diagnosis and Mrs Davis was admitted to the acute medical ward. She was complaining of an intense headache and that the light hurt her eyes. She was obviously very frightened, continually seeking reassurance from the nurses that she would be all right.

She was moved into a single room with the blinds drawn to reduce the light and to allow quietness, but the nurse assigned to care for her stayed with her.

The doctor explained to Mrs Davis what he thought had caused her sudden headache and that she was to be kept under close observation. He also explained this to Mr Davis and added that his wife was at great risk of having a further haemorrhage so once the cause was identified surgery would probably be indicated. Mr Davis was visibly shaken by the devastating news. The ward sister sat with Mr Davis whilst he had a cup of tea and again went over what the doctor had said. She reassured him that, although surgery to the brain was not without great risk, a high proportion of patients did extremely well after surgery following a subarachnoid haemorrhage.

Analgesia was prescribed and given, care being taken to give adequate pain relief without the risk of altering the patient's level of consciousness, as this may obscure the assessment of the patient (whether her condition was stable or deteriorating). Drugs which may be used are Codeine Phosphate or Dihydrocodeine. If the pain is not controlled it is impossible for the patient to rest and this is essential following a subarachnoid haemorrhage.

To confirm the diagnosis of subarachnoid haemorrhage a lumbar puncture was performed.

The cerebrospinal fluid was uniformly bloodstained confirming the diagnosis.

Following a subarachnoid haemorrhage enforced rest for several days is essential to allow the damaged blood vessel to heal by the formation of a blood clot. Any exertion is likely to dislodge the clot and result in further bleeding and even death. Drugs such as Tranexamic Acid may be given to prevent the blood clot from being broken down thus rendering it more stable.

To avoid increased pressure on the damaged blood vessel Mrs Davis was nursed flat in bed with one pillow, but allowed to turn from side to side. The number of pillows was gradually increased over several days until she was sitting upright. During this time she was allowed to use the commode at the side of the bed with constant supervision as this is less likely to cause strain on the cerebral blood vessels than when perched on a bedpan. The nurse assigned to care for her attended to all her activities of daily living, including washing and assisting with meals.

As the headache came under control and the nausea subsided Mrs Davis became less anxious. Her husband and children visited every day and brought her up-to-date with news of

A lumbar puncture is the passing of a special needle, under aseptic conditions, into the subarachnoid space of the spinal cord, between either the third and fourth, or fourth and fifth lumbar vertebrae. A specimen of cerebrospinal fluid (CSF) is obtained and the pressure of the fluid may also be estimated.

Aneurysm The dilatation of a weakened section of an artery, most commonly occurring in the cerebral circulation or the aorta.

their local community. The regular contact with her family helped to reassure Mrs Davis that they were managing well at home.

In order that the cause of the subarachnoid haemorrhage could be identified it was arranged for Mrs Davis to have an angiogram of her cerebral blood vessels. This confirmed the presence of an aneurysm.

Cerebral angiography is the injection of a radio-opaque dye into the cerebral circulation, followed by X-rays which demonstrate the cerebral circulation. The injection may be made directly into the carotid artery or via the femoral, vertebral or axillary artery. This X-ray procedure is used to pin-point the site of bleeding in subarachnoid haemorrhage, or the presence of a cerebral tumour. It is usually performed under general anaesthesia. Regular observation of the injection site is essential following the X-ray as there is a risk of haemorrhage.

As there is always the possibility that once a cerebral aneurysm has ruptured it can happen again, Mrs Davis was transferred to the neuro-surgical unit where she had the aneurysm clipped to avoid further problems. This operation is not without great risk but four weeks afterwards Mrs Davis visited the medical ward again to thank the staff for the care she had received. She had a very slight weakness of her left arm and leg but said this was improving every day and she was confident that, with regular physiotherapy, normal use would return and she would soon be back at school again.

The following aspects of care are common for all patients following a subarachnoid haemorrhage:

Note immediately any change in the patient's neurological state as this may indicate further bleeding.

Note reaction of pupils to light, level of consciousness, pulse, blood pressure, movement of limbs, every hour. Report any changes to the doctor immediately. If these observations remain stable they may be taken less frequently.

Ensure the patient remains at rest to enable the damaged blood vessel to become sealed by a stable blood clot.	Nurse flat with one pillow. The nurse must take over all activities of daily living for the patient.
Relief of pain, to ensure the patient is able to rest.	Give the patient adequate and regular analgesia, and assess its effectiveness. If not effective discuss increase in dose or change of analgesia with the doctor.
Avoid strain and exertion which may dislodge the blood clot.	Allow to use commode at the bedside with a nurse in attendance. Avoid constipation.

Safety – of patients, visitors, staff

Procedure – nursing
Established methods of carrying out nursing actions which are uniformly practised. They are usually laid down in a procedure manual, either as a rigid procedure or as a series of principles.

Policy – nursing
Plans drawn up locally by nurse managers, covering many aspects of nursing. The aim of set policies is to safeguard both patients and staff.

Throughout your nursing career you must bear in mind all aspects of safety – not only for the patients but for visitors, colleagues and your-self. This means adhering to procedures and policies as laid down by your employing health authority and taught in the school of nursing. If you feel unable to follow procedures and policies because of inadequate equipment or because some members of the ward team dis-courage you, have the courage to discuss this with the ward sister or charge nurse.

It is imperative that you follow the lifting techniques you have been taught, to avoid injury to the patient, yourself or your col-leagues. If you are uncertain about the proper methods for lifting patients, ask a trained member of the ward team.

Always dispose of 'sharps' such as needles, blades, etc. in the special container provided, to avoid injuring unsuspecting persons. Soiled dressings must also be disposed of in the proper manner.

In order to protect patients from injury close observation may be essential, especially those with a suicidal tendency or those who are confused or hyperactive. The effective use of safety aids, when indicated, may be useful in the prevention of injury.

Never leave equipment or patients' belongings, e.g. slippers, in such a place that they may constitute a hazard for either patients, visitors or staff. Water or lotions spilt on the floor constitute a danger and should be removed immediately.

If a patient or visitor to the ward tells you they have injured themselves you *must* report this to the nurse in charge of the ward straight-away, who will then take the appropriate action.

If you injure yourself whilst on duty you *must* also report this to the nurse in charge. A formal report will be written on the appropriate form and you will be examined by a doctor, depending on hospital policy. This is usually the doctor in the Accident and Emergency Department or in the Occupational Health Department.

No accident to either patients, visitors or staff should go unreported as there may be legal implications at a later date.

8 Ensuring a restful atmosphere

What are the effects of lack of rest and sleep?

Lethargy
Irritability, especially with loved ones
Inability to cope with the uncertainty and stress of illness
Lack of interest in own care
Lack of independence
Decrease in self-respect and self-esteem

Rest and sleep promote recovery, and aiding rest is an essential aspect of nursing care. All patients need to have a good night's rest, but the amount of sleep will vary from patient to patient and it is important to be aware of the individual's normal sleep pattern.

The amount of bed rest required in the day also varies and is determined by many personal factors as well as by the medical condition.

Some of the factors which will determine the amount of bed rest required during the day:

Reason for being in hospital – after a myocardial infarction rest is indicated, but less rest is required during rehabilitation following a cerebrovascular accident
Age
Other disabilities – a patient with an arthritic hip may not be able to lie in bed for any length of time even if indicated by his medical condition
How ill the patient feels
Pyrexia
Severe pain

Pyrexia A rise above normal (36.8°C or 98.4°F) of body temperature.

In order to rest the patient does not necessarily need to be in bed but in the position most comfortable for relaxing and breathing. This may be in an easy chair. Indeed, many patients are more comfortable and able to relax and sleep in a reclining easy chair, rather than in bed.

The caring, understanding nurse can help the patient to rest and sleep *without* immediately resorting to tranquillisers and sleeping tablets.

What may prevent a patient from resting and sleeping?

Change of environment and loss of familiar surroundings
Depressive illness leading to early waking
Being separated from family and friends
Loss of independence
Being with strangers
Worry, fear and anxiety
Pain
Too cold/too warm
Noise
Light at night
Change of bed
Uncomfortable bed

How can we aid sleep and rest?

ensure a quiet, peaceful and calming atmosphere:
  quiet demeanour
  quiet shoes
  careful, gentle handling of patient
  quietness of speech and no shouting
  careful use of equipment
  not allowing doors to bang

ensure comfort:
  bed or chair
  adequate pillows
  adequate blankets
  not too hot or too cold
  not hungry or thirsty

relief of pain and discomfort

relief of anxiety and fear:
  keep patient fully informed
  explain use of special equipment
  involve social worker if indicated
  ensure family are coping

allow family and friends access

The complications of bed rest were discussed in Chapter 4 and it is very apparent that resting in bed is loaded with potential dangers. In a medical setting very few of the patients will be required to stay in bed for any length of time except for the following special cases.

The unconscious patient is kept at rest, flat in bed and in the lateral position to ensure an adequate airway.

Patients with severe heart failure need to be kept at rest in the early stages of treatment to allow the pumping mechanism of the heart to be more effective, so that fluid retained in the tissues may be reabsorbed and excreted via the kidneys.

It is better for patients in severe pain to be encouraged to rest in bed or any position they find comfortable until their pain is controlled. The patient who has had a myocardial infarction must rest to avoid undue strain on the heart. By and large, bed rest is enforced if there is a danger of exacerbating the patient's medi-

Oedema
Excessive accumulation of fluid in the tissue spaces.

cal problem, but the golden rule is to keep the patient in bed for as short a time as possible in order to reduce to a minimum the risk of complications.

You will be guided by the trained nurses as to how long a patient is to be in bed. Unless otherwise indicated, patients having special treatment such as blood transfusions, intravenous infusions, bladder drainage, are not confined to bed.

Patients who need to stay in bed may become very frustrated because of the loss of independence. They may take the law into their own hands and get up. This tends to occur if the patient has not been told the reasons for resting. Careful explanation to the patient, therefore, is essential, and this may need to be reinforced again and again.

You will need much tact and courtesy with the patient who keeps asking 'Why can't I get up when I want to?' to explain the reason for a gradual return to normality. Some patients who have had a myocardial infarction and feel better once the pain has subsided, may find it particularly difficult to rely on other people for their needs.

HISTORY

Meet Mr Brown who has had a Myocardial Infarction

Mr Brown was a 56 year old painter and decorator. Whilst at work he suddenly developed crushing, central chest pain which radiated up into his throat and down both arms and a strangling sensation. His colleague called an ambulance and he was brought into the casualty department where a diagnosis of myocardial infarction was made.

A myocardial infarction (or heart attack) is death of part of the heart muscle due to occlusion of the blood supply and therefore of oxygen. It is caused by atheroma (fat deposits within the walls of the coronary artery concerned). The artery becomes narrowed and finally occluded by a blood clot. The onset is usually sudden, with severe crushing central chest pain, which is persistent, even at rest.

Many patients have previously had angina, pain occurring at first on exertion, caused by a reduction in the blood supply to the heart muscle but not complete obstruction.

Right atrium

Right coronary artery

Right ventricle

Infarcted heart muscle

Left coronary artery

Left ventricle

Site of occlusion

NURSING CARE

Mr Brown was immediately transferred to the acute medical ward after being given an intravenous injection of Diamorphine to relieve his pain. (In most large hospitals there is a Coronary Care Unit where patients like Mr Brown are admitted for the first 48 hours. This is because complications following a heart attack are more likely to occur during this period of time. The staff in the Coronary Care Unit are specially trained to observe for, and treat, any abnormalities as they occur in order to try and prevent life threatening complications from developing.)

On arrival to the ward Mr Brown was pale but sleepy, and free from pain. He was accompanied by his wife who appeared very anxious although in full control. He was settled into bed and attached to a cardiac monitor, the significance of the machine being explained to him first. The doctor arranged for an ECG straight away.

A cardiac monitor is a special machine which picks up the electrical activity of the heart via electrodes placed on the chest. Any abnormal heart rhythms can be identified immediately and treated accordingly. A constant check can be made of the heart's activity.

An ECG (electro-cardiograph) is a graph which demonstrates the heart's electrical activity which causes contraction of the heart muscle. It is performed by using a special machine with leads attached to the body by means of electrodes. It is used by the doctor to confirm or aid the diagnosis of heart disease.

A normal heart beat

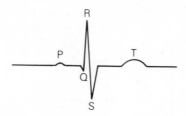

P – contraction of atria
QRS – contraction of ventricles

T – repolarisation of heart muscles – ready for the next beat

Whilst the doctor was examining Mr Brown the ward sister talked to his wife, explaining that, if the diagnosis of a heart attack was confirmed, Mr Brown would be in hospital for about 7–10 days and he would need a period of 8–12 weeks convalescence. The significance of the cardiac monitor was explained and also the fact that Mr Brown had had an injection to relieve his pain and that this had made him drowsy.

The sister gently told Mrs Brown that the first 48 hours were the most crucial, as this was the time when cardiac complications were most likely to occur, but that he was being kept under close observation and at rest. This involved him being bedbathed by the nurse, but he was allowed to sit in a chair just whilst his bed was made. He was also allowed out of bed to use the commode. Steps were taken to prevent the complications of bedrest, as described in Chapter 4.

The nurse assigned to care for Mr Brown observed his cardiac monitor at least every hour, looking for any change in rhythm which, if observed, would be reported to the doctor immediately. The presence of the cardiac monitor seemed to reassure Mr Brown. The nurse also measured his blood pressure every 4

Hypertension
The elevation of the blood pressure above normal. Normal blood pressure varies with age and depends mainly on peripheral resistance of the arteries and the circulating volume within them.

hours to ensure that hypotension or hypertension was quickly noted.

After 48 hours the cardiac monitor was discontinued and Mr Brown sat out of bed each day for an increasing length of time. A bowl was now placed at his bedside and he was allowed to wash himself with assistance by the nurse if needed. On the sixth day he was permitted to walk around his bed and then as far as the toilet.

Coping with constipation adds strain on the heart so a careful check was made on Mr Brown's bowel activity. As he had not had his bowels opened on the third day he was given a mild aperient which had the desired effect.

The gradual increase in Mr Brown's activity was planned in such a way as to reduce any adverse strain to his damaged heart muscle, and was carefully explained to him.

In the initial stages of his admission it was ascertained that Mr and Mrs Brown would be able to manage financially until Mr Brown was able to resume work. They had a son who was working but living at home and Mrs Brown had a part-time job.

Mr Brown was allowed home on the tenth day and his wife fetched him in the car. He was told to gradually increase his activities over the next six weeks, until he resumed his normal lifestyle.

Advice to patients following a myocardial infarction:

Avoid strain on the heart – no lifting as in gardening, no sudden exertion as in squash.

Have plenty of rest, initially resting in the afternoons.

Do a little more each day.

If pain or breathlessness occurs reduce activity a little.

If pain or breathlessness persists contact your doctor immediately.

Do not return to work until advised by your doctor.

Do not drive for about 2 months.

Stop smoking.

Avoid becoming overweight and eat fat sparingly.

Booklets issued by the British Heart Foundation are available giving basic information about the effects of a heart attack and advising on future lifestyle. If used they should also be backed up by discussion with the doctor and nursing staff, and it is essential to check the patient's understanding before he is discharged home.

The following points may be common to all patients following a myocardial infarction:

Relief of pain to ensure rest	Nurse patient in position most comfortable for him. Give analgesia at regular intervals as prescribed. Inform doctor if it is not effective or if pain persists.
Early identification of abnormal cardiac rhythm (arrhythmias) so that they may be treated immediately	Nurse patient connected to cardiac monitor. Observe monitor at least every hour and note heart rate and rhythm. Inform doctor of any adverse changes.
Risk of developing heart failure and fluid retention, if heart's pumping mechanism is affected	Observe and report any signs of increasing dyspnoea, or oedema of ankles or sacrum. Maintain an accurate record of fluid intake and output.
 Avoid straining the already damaged heart muscle, allowing it time to heal	Encourage patient to rest. Relief of pain. Activities of daily living to be carried out by the nurse for the first 48 hours. Gradually increase activity over next 4–5 days until patient is washing self and able to walk to toilet and washroom. Avoid constipation. Reduce anxiety by allowing patient to express anxieties, and explain aims and plan of care, use of special equipment and tests.

Following a myocardial infarction some patients experience no further problems. Others may develop the following:

1   Recurrent infarctions
2   Cardiac failure – will need to take diuretic drugs (which cause the kidneys to excrete sodium and water e.g. Frusemide)
3   Arrhythmias e.g. atrial fibrillation for which Digoxin may be given
4   Heart block – may need insertion of a pacemaker.
5   Angina – Glyceryl Trinitrate is given to prevent or treat attacks of angina.

Cardiac arrest

Following a myocardial infarction some patients may develop arrhythmias (electrical disturbance of the heart muscle) which can cause the heart to stop beating suddenly. This is known as a *cardiac arrest* and immediate action must be taken otherwise the patient will die.

Signs of cardiac arrest
Loss of consciousness
Gasping or absent respirations
Dilated pupils
Absence of major pulses
Twitching
Cyanosis

Action to be taken
Act immediately
Ensure airway is clear e.g. remove false teeth
Lie patient flat on firm surface
Thump chest at sternum
Summon help – shout or ring emergency bell

1st nurse
Cardiac massage – compress lower third of sternum approximately 1.5 inches with heel of hand using squeezing action, at approximately 70 times per minute.

A bone marrow puncture is the aspiration of bone marrow from the sternum or iliac crest using a special needle and a syringe. The bone marrow fluid is placed on microscope slides for examination. It is an uncomfortable and sometimes painful procedure. The examination of the bone marrow is a valuable aid to diagnosis in patients with diseases of the blood and bone marrow. During the procedure the nurse's role is to reassure the patient.

A blood transfusion is the administration of blood, either whole blood or packed cells – plasma is removed to leave a high concentration of red cells in a reduced amount of plasma – via the venous system.

During the transfusion the patient is carefully observed for any adverse reactions to the blood such as tachycardia, pyrexia, rigors and back pain.

2nd nurse

Insert airway into mouth, and using Ambubag attached to oxygen supply and face mask of appropriate size placed over nose and mouth, squeeze air into lungs.

Sequence: Cardiac massage 10–15 compressions

Artificial respiration 2–3 inflations

Ensure a nurse has raised the cardiac arrest alarm.

In most hospitals a team of doctors will quickly arrive at the ward once the alarm has been raised, and the senior doctor will then direct the resuscitation procedure.

Witnessing and taking part in the cardiac arrest procedure can be a very frightening experience, even for trained nurses. It is also frightening for the other patients so never forget them – they will need care and support and someone to talk to. If possible it is better to move the other patients to the day room. Those who cannot be moved should not be left alone whilst another patient is being resuscitated.

Anaemia

Any person during illness will feel tired to a greater or lesser degree and will require a certain amount of rest. Any anaemic patient will be especially tired and may need help with the normal activities of daily living.

Patients being investigated for anaemia will require a full blood count and may also need a bone marrow puncture.

One of the treatments used for patients with anaemia is blood transfusion.

Nursing the patient who is dying

Although dying and death still tend to be taboo subjects in Western society, there is a growing tendency to talk about them more openly, and the media – both the press and television – are devoting more time to it.

Dying and death must be talked about openly, if nurses are to cope with it and be of support and comfort to patients and relatives. Nurses who find they cannot cope, or who feel they get no support from the trained nurses on the ward, tend to appear cold and aloof and give the impression of not caring.

In the medical ward you will be involved with patients who die suddenly, i.e. they collapse and die within minutes, or are admitted in a dying state and death occurs soon after, and with patients whose death is preceded by a period of degeneration, which is termed the terminal stage of the disease, or terminal illness.

In the United Kingdom the major causes of death are heart disease, cancer and stroke, diseases all encountered in the medical ward.

Malignant disease (cancer) is the disease most usually associated with dying and death, but other diseases can be equally fatal. A patient making an uneventful recovery from a myocardial infarction may develop a further more serious infarction or cardiac arrhythmia and die. Someone receiving treatment for a transient loss of consciousness may have a stroke and die. A patient with congestive cardiac failure may be resistant to treatment and gradually worsen and die.

Cancer develops when the normal control mechanism of cellular division is lost. A mass of tissue – a tumour – forms, which extends beyond the normal confines of the organ. Cancer cells, also referred to as malignant cells, have the ability to spread to other parts of the body and cause further damage. They spread either directly, or via the blood or lymphatic system.

Occasionally patients receiving treatment for common medically orientated diseases may develop complications whilst in the ward and die:

e.g. diabetes mellitus → ketoacidosis
    asthma   → respiratory failure
    hypertension   → cerebrovascular
                            accident

Most of these diseases, except cancer, have been discussed elsewhere in this book.

Nearly all malignant tumours are fatal unless treated. Treatment includes radiotherapy, hormone therapy, cytotoxic drug therapy and surgery, and often involves more than one of these treatments.

Dying versus Cardiac Arrest

Many nurses find it difficult to differentiate between cardiac arrest and dying.

Cardiac arrest is the sudden cessation of effective heart action and therefore of blood flow to the brain; however, sometimes the patient can be resuscitated and not die. Everyone who dies has a cardiac arrest, though this may be secondary to other causes of death. Before resuscitative measures are begun (see Chapter 8) it is essential to know whether the patient should be resuscitated.

Patients with progressive disease may respond to having their symptoms treated as they appear, in order to be more comfortable and perhaps gain a slight extension of life expectancy, but in whom the cardiac arrest procedure is not contemplated. For example a patient with leukaemia who has failed to respond to cytotoxic chemotherapy and is terminally ill may be given platelet or blood transfusions to stop bleeding and to correct anaemia, thereby making the patient more comfortable.

Leukaemia The excessive production of abnormal white cells by the bone marrow. It is one form of cancer of the blood.

If communication on the ward is clear and effective you will usually know which patients are dying and with whom the policy is to keep them comfortable and pain-free. Obviously there will be times when you are not sure whether to instigate the cardiac arrest procedure, and the golden rule must be, *if in doubt, attempt to resuscitate*.

Care of the Dying Patient

The aim of care for the dying patient is to ensure that the dying process is peaceful, pain-free and dignified. This means that all symptoms must be understood, anticipated and controlled.

It goes without saying that these patients must be treated as individuals in the context of their families and social background, approaching them as normal human beings, and involving them in the decision-making affecting their care.

The symptoms and signs of terminal illness following may arise during the terminal stages of a patient's illness, but not all will necessarily occur: fear and anxiety, pain, nausea and vomiting, anorexia, weight loss, breathlessness, incontinence, constipation or diarrhoea, changes in physical appearance, confusion, insomnia, fungating lesions. Some of these, such as nausea, insomnia, breathlessness and incontinence, should be treated as described earlier in the book, together with the appropriate drugs, following discussion with the doctor.

Fungating lesions are treated with the appropriate local applications and dressings. If an offensive odour is present, the use of dressings such as carbon pads may reduce it.

Changes in physical appearance will cause the patient distress, and reinforces the need to treat the patient as an individual and to decline from making comment unless the patient does so. Physical changes can also be very distressing for the relatives.

Fear and anxiety. Patients react to awareness of impending death differently. Those patients who do not know, but who suspect, may be tense and stressed. Once their fears are confirmed they are often relieved, and accept the situation.

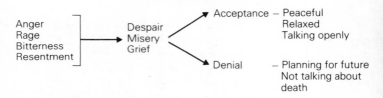

Many patients in the terminal stages of a disease are aware that they are dying, even though it may not have been discussed with them. Some will talk openly about it, others will not, either to deny impending death to themselves or in an attempt to protect their loved ones.

It is important that you look for cues, signalling that the patient wants to talk. Some patients will openly discuss their fears and anxieties for themselves and for their family. Others may hint with a variety of statements, such as:

'I don't think the treatment has worked, Nurse.'

'I don't seem to be getting any better.'

'Mr Jones has gone home today. I don't think I will ever go home again.'

Always try to ask an open-ended question (one where the patient has to elaborate) rather than a closed question (when the patient can answer either 'Yes' or 'No') e.g. 'What makes you think that?'

If a patient asks 'Am I going to die, Nurse?' your answer will depend on the stage of the patient's illness:

'No, you are not going to die'	Patient who is not dying
'Hopefully not yet. We are trying this new line of treatment so you must continue to be positive and hope that the treatment will be effective.'	Patient who has a potentially fatal illness
'What do you understand by your condition? What have you been told?'	Patient who is dying
'I don't know, but I will fetch sister to talk to you straightaway as she knows much more about your illness than I do.'	Patient who is dying

It is vital that patients feel they can express their anxieties and fears. Allowing them time is of paramount importance. Even if you are busy try not to look rushed, but sit with a patient if you anticipate he or she wants to talk.

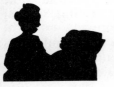

Never appear casual or unconcerned, even if this is your way of coping. If you cannot deal with the questions, anxieties or fears the patient expresses, refer to a trained nurse immediately and tell the patient what you are doing. If you feel out of your depth never disappear leaving the patient alone and unsure of what is happening. Talk to sister and explain your fears and anxieties after she has spoken to the patient.

Pain. Many people are afraid that death will be painful, but with modern drugs and a sensitive approach by both nurses and doctors it is usually possible to completely control pain.

Examples of analgesia (pain-relieving drugs) used in terminal care:

Aspirin
Dihydrocodeine
Dextromoramide
Diamorphine

During your day-to-day contact with the patient you have an ideal opportunity to assess the effectiveness of the analgesia, noticing whether pain occurs at rest, on movement or not at all. You should inform the senior nurse of your observations.

The art of good pain control is to anticipate the pain and to give the drugs before the pain occurs. Usually this means giving them at regular intervals rather than on demand, depending on the drug used and the individual's needs and wishes.

HISTORY

Meet Jane who dies following acute leukaemia

Jane was 39 years old and had three children, a 19 year old daughter from her first marriage, a 6 year old son and 4 year old daughter from her second marriage. She and her husband were obviously extremely devoted to one another and they were a very close family.

Jane had been treated for acute leukaemia for four years, and relapsed nine months ago. The disease continued unabated despite several courses of different very strong cytotoxic drugs.

Jane had always taken a keen interest in her treatment and progress and despite the relapse managed to maintain a positive approach. Following each course of drugs she would nervously wait for news of any improvement in her blood or bone marrow tests; she was increasingly aware that treatments available to her were becoming fewer.

The consultant told her, as the last available treatment was commenced, that if it was unsuccessful there was little else he could offer, but at the moment there was still a slight chance.

On completion of the treatment Jane realised that she was no better, and seemed to be gradually accepting the inevitable outcome. She talked to the sister and nurses about how she felt and seemed to find their presence and understanding comforting and supportive.

The next day Jane's husband was seen by the consultant and told that Jane would die within the next few weeks as nothing had worked. He was obviously distressed, although half expecting this news.

His immediate reaction was that once he was composed he himself would tell Jane as they had always shared everything. The ward sister made him a cup of tea and sat with him whilst he talked about his sadness, not only for himself, but for the children. He was going to tell his step-daughter when he got home. He was not bitter, but grateful for the happiness they had had together.

Sister provided a further tray of tea and ensured that Jane and her husband had complete privacy. They talked and cried together and later appeared quite composed.

From then on Jane talked openly about dying. She expressed sadness and regret that she would not see her young children grow up but thankful that they would be well cared for. She was also sad that she would not see her eldest daughter get married.

The hospital chaplain gave her a lot of support and her faith increased. She talked about symptoms that might arise and was constantly reassured that these would be controlled. She often said that she was glad she had been in the same room as Pam when she had died. Pam had also had acute leukaemia and they had been very friendly. Jane felt reassured because she had witnessed at first hand the kindness and care both Pam and her family had received, and that Pam had died peacefully and free from pain.

Jane began to develop bone pain which was counteracted with doses of Diamorphine. The nurses kept a close watch on Jane to ensure that the pain was controlled. The sister discussed her pain control each day and more often if indicated, with the doctor, the dose of the drug being increased as necessary.

Jane died peacefully one afternoon a few days later, with her husband and daughter at her bedside, holding her hands.

Care of the Family in Terminal Illness

If a patient is dying it is vital that the family are aware and have access as often as they and the patient wish, with the opportunity to stay at the bedside. Encourage the patient to be as mobile and active as possible.

Contact and communication with the family is equally as important as with the patient. In some cases, involve them in the patient's care (as long as this is what the patient and relative wish). This can include helping to give drinks or with washing.

Allow time for the family to talk and express their fears and anxieties; this will make them realise that the nursing staff care for them and understand how they feel. They may want to talk about the patient, personal characteristics, accomplishments and achievements. Do not feel embarrassed if they cry or show anger. Do inform sister or staff nurse how the relatives are reacting to this extremely stressful situation.

Care of the Family at the Time of Death

Nursing is said to be a caring profession but the Health Service Ombudsman receives many complaints about the way bereaved relatives are treated in hospital. This has resulted in health authorities being requested by the Government to draw up guidelines for staff on how to deal with bereaved relatives.

Whether death is sudden or expected the effect on the family can be just as devastating. Grief, disbelief, anger, resentment or relief may be demonstrated.

Relatives need time to take in what has happened and a cup of tea and a comfortable seat, in privacy, gives an opportunity for the reality of the situation to be slowly assimilated. Rushing them off the ward is callous and thoughtless. Many relatives appreciate being allowed time alone with the body. Seeing the body after death often makes the death a reality and a little easier to eventually accept.

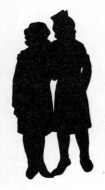

The relatives will often want to talk, about the person who has died, or about the practical things they need to do, or about irrelevant matters. They should, to a certain extent, be allowed to dictate the conversation. The nurse will be more supportive if she lends an ear, or a comforting hand, rather than making thoughtless comments such as 'Don't be upset', or 'Don't cry'.

Involving other Health Care Workers

Other health care workers are available to give support and also practical help to both patient and family. Sister or staff nurse will liaise with them but if you feel a certain health care worker may be able to make a useful contribution to a patient or relative, suggest this to sister. Health care workers include: social worker, chaplain, physiotherapist, occupational therapist, dietician, community nurse (if the patient is to be nursed at home).

Care of the Body

If you have never seen a dead body before you may feel very apprehensive and possibly afraid. You will find that the patient, perhaps white or slightly mottled, looks asleep.

Once the doctor has certified death and it has been ensured that the family have spent as much time as they feel necessary with the body, it is washed and prepared for the mortuary, according to the local nursing procedure. This is known as last offices. The body should be treated with respect throughout. In some hospitals it is the policy to leave the body undisturbed for about an hour before carrying out the last offices, once the body has been straightened.

Care of Other Patients

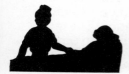

If the patient has died in a room with other patients they should be told what has happened. On the other hand, if the patient has been in a single room patients on the ward may inquire about his or her welfare, and should always be told the truth. If lied to, they will eventually find out anyway, and you may well have lost their trust in the process. Once aware, other patients may cry, and must be allowed to do so without embarrassment. They too, will need comfort and support from you.

10 Leaving the medical ward

Patients you have met and cared for and come
to like and respect will be moving on; patients
on an acute medical ward are not usually

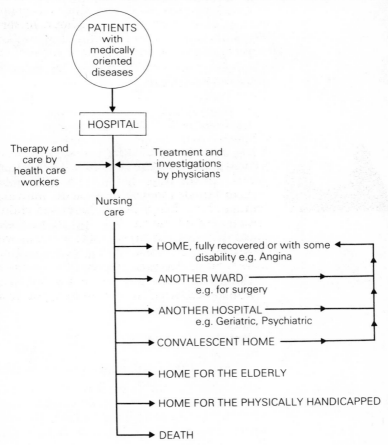

static, even if a small proportion wait many months before going home or moving to another hospital. You will help to prepare them for discharge or transfer.

When a patient moves from the ward there are several matters which must be attended to first, usually by a senior nurse but you may also be involved:

Discharge of patient
*Inform patient
*Inform relatives
*Arrange transport
Outpatients' appointment
Transport for appointment
Inform health care workers
Arrange tablets, dressings
Special instructions e.g. steroid card
District nurse visits
Letter for district nurse (written by a nurse)
*Letter for general practitioner (written by a doctor)
Medical certificates
*Clothes
Valuables
*Inform admissions office
*Complete nursing records

Transfer of patient
*Inform patient
*Inform relatives
*Arrange transport
Nurse escort
*Inform receiving ward
Inform health care workers
May need tablets
*Transfer letters from doctor/nurse
Valuables
*Clothes
*Check if to take notes, X-rays, and inform medical records office
*Inform admissions office
*Complete nursing records

Those marked * will apply for every patient.

Before any patient is discharged home it is vital to ensure that the social conditions are suitable, e.g. if a patient has had a stroke and is unable to negotiate stairs, that there is a bed and commode downstairs, or if a patient lives alone, that they have a key to get in and a supply of food is available. This is why it is essential to involve other health care workers before discharge as well as the relatives.

Patients who are to be discharged or transferred from the ward may react in different ways. Remember that for some patients it may mean leaving newly made friends – both other patients and staff – to go home to be alone, with only the milkman calling each day.

For those to be transferred it will mean having to meet yet more new people and trying to build up a relationship with them, so do not forget that both discharge and transfer can be extremely stressful times for the patient.

The patient may be excited, hyperactive, apprehensive, nervous or depressed and therefore needs help to prepare for the move. It is essential that patient and family are aware of the impending move and they may ask you for further information (e.g. often they think patients must go home in the morning). In most hospitals the time of discharge will depend on availability of transport. If you are not sure, however, refer any queries to the nurse in charge.

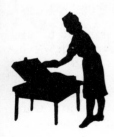

On the day of discharge or transfer, once the patient has had a wash he or she may need help with dressing. Remember that after several days in hospital getting dressed can be an ordeal, especially for the elderly. Help with packing personal belongings is often much appreciated – an excited or nervous patient often leaves things behind so do check the locker, wardrobe and bed area.

Usually the patient will not need to vacate the bed until it is time to leave the ward but this will depend on ward or hospital policy.

As the patient is about to leave, ensure that he or she has:

All personal belongings

Appointment card

Tablets (and understands what they are for and when to take them)

Written instructions for medication for future reference

Dressings

Letters

Special appliances

If the patient is being taken home by relatives make sure that they are able to get to the exit without difficulty.

You, too, may soon be moving on to another ward and a different type of nursing experience – surgical, gynaecological, ophthalmic, orthopaedic, paediatric, geriatric or psychiatric nursing. There are, however, many nursing skills and principles of care you have practised and developed on the medical ward which you will be able to apply to many varied nursing situations throughout your training.

Attitudes you have formed during your medical experience will continue to influence your approach to patients, patient care, relatives and colleagues. Your attitude, therefore, as a member of a caring profession should be one of care, concern, compassion and empathy.

Always aim to give a high standard of care and, even when the going gets tough, never lower your standard but still strive for it, even if you do not always get there.

If you are a member of a ward team where this quotation applies you can feel that you are involved in giving care of a high standard.

An assessment of the best standard of care in a ward is a ward where: patients are comfortable patients and staff are happy patients, relatives and nurses feel fully informed about what is happening patients get well quickly or die peacefully and with dignity.

Matthews, 1982

Further Reading

ANTHONY, C. P. 1983. *A Textbook of Anatomy and Physiology*, 11th ed. St. Louis: C. V. Mosby Co.

BLOOM, A. 1981. *Toohey's Medicine for Nurses*, 13th ed. Edinburgh: Churchill Livingstone.

BOORE, J. 1978. *Prescription for Recovery*. Edinburgh: Churchill Livingstone/Royal College of Nursing.

BOOTH, J. A. (Ed). 1982. *Nurse's Handbook of Investigations*. Lippincott Nursing Series. London: Harper and Row Ltd.

BRUNER, L. S. & SUDDARTH, D. S. 1983. *The Lippincott Manual of Medical-Surgical Nursing* (3 vols.). Lippincott Nursing Series. London: Harper and Row Ltd.

CHILMAN, A. M. & THOMAS, M. (Eds). 1981. *Understanding Nursing Care*, 2nd ed. Edinburgh: Churchill Livingstone.

GREEN, J. H. 1976. *An Introduction to Human Physiology*. Oxford: Oxford University Press.

HAYWARD, J. 1975. *Information – A Prescription Against Pain*. London: Royal College of Nursing.

HEATH, J. & LAW, G. M. 1982. *Nursing Process – What is it!* Sheffield: NHS Learning Resources Unit.

HENDERSON, V. 1968. *Basic Principles of Nursing Care*. Geneva: International Council of Nurses.

HENNEY, C. R., DOW, R. J., MACCONNACHIE, A. M. & CROOKS, J. 1982. *Drugs in Nursing Practice. A Handbook*. Edinburgh: Churchill Livingstone.

HOUSTON, J. C., JOINER, C. L. & TROUNCE, J. R. 1985. *A Short Textbook of Medicine*, 8th ed. Sevenoaks: Hodder and Stoughton Ltd.

MACLEOD, J. (Ed). 1981. *Davidson's Principles and Practice of Medicine*, 13th ed. Edinburgh: Churchill Livingstone.

MATTHEWS, A. 1982. *In Charge of the Ward*. Oxford: Blackwell Scientific Publications.

POLETTI, R. 1983. In: 'NT Week', *Nursing Times*, Nov 30, p20.

ROPER, N. 1982. *Principles of Nursing*. Edinburgh: Churchill Livingstone.

SCHOLES, M. E., WILSON, J. L. & MACRAE, S. 1982. *Handbook of Nursing Procedures*. Oxford: Blackwell Scientific Publications.

WILSON-BARNETT, J. 1979. *Stress in Hospital – Patients' Psychological Reactions to Illness and Health Care*. Edinburgh: Churchill Livingstone.

WILSON-BARNETT, J. 1978. 'Patients' emotional responses to barium X-rays.' *Journal of Advanced Nursing*, 3(1), 37–46.

INDEX